FOREWORD BY Charles R. Cantor, MD, DABSM,
Medical Director, Penn Sleep Centers

365 WAYS TO GET A GOOD NIGHT'S SLEEP

Ronald L. Kotler, MD, DABSM,
Medical Director, Pennsylvania Hos
and Maryann

A adams

Avon, Massachusetts

D0451825

Published by
Adams Media, a division of F+W Media, Inc.
57 Littlefield Street, Avon, MA 02322. U.S.A.
www.adamsmedia.com

ISBN 10: 1-60550-101-8
ISBN 13: 978-1-60550-101-7

Printed in the United States of America.

JIHGFEDCBA

Library of Congress Cataloging-in-Publication Data
is available from the publisher.

This publication is designed to provide accurate and authoritative information with regard to the subject matter covered. It is sold with the understanding that the publisher is not engaged in rendering legal, accounting, or other professional advice. If legal advice or other expert assistance is required, the services of a competent professional person should be sought.

—From a *Declaration of Principles* jointly adopted by a Committee of the American Bar Association and a Committee of Publishers and Associations

Many of the designations used by manufacturers and sellers to distinguish their product are claimed as trademarks. Where those designations appear in this book and Adams Media was aware of a trademark claim, the designations have been printed with initial capital letters.

365 Ways to Get a Good Night's Sleep is intended as a reference volume only, not as a medical manual. In light of the complex, individual, and specific nature of health problems, this book is not intended to replace professional medical advice. The ideas, procedures, and suggestions in this book are intended to supplement, not replace, the advice of a trained medical professional. Consult your physician before adopting the suggestions in this book, as well as about any condition that may require diagnosis or medical attention. The author and publisher disclaim any liability arising directly or indirectly from the use of this book.

This book is available at quantity discounts for bulk purchases.
For information, please call 1-800-289-0963.

To my wife and soul mate, Jane Kotler;
She is always by my side.

To my children, Jennifer Kotler, Rachel Slama, and Drew Kotler;
They have taught me the meaning of unconditional love.

To my parents, Milton Kotler and Marion Kotler;
They have provided me with opportunity.

To my siblings, Kenneth Kotler, Mark Kotler, and Sherry Greenberger;

To my best friend, Dr. David Sherer;

And to all my patients, who have entrusted me with their
greatest gift, the gift of life.

—*Ron Kotler*

To Mom, Karl, and Jim, who ease my mind
so I can get a good night's sleep,

and to Patti, David, Karen, and Judith who provide me with
comfy places to put my head when I'm on the road.

—*Maryann Karinch*

Contents

Acknowledgments

Thirty years ago, I entered medical school with a thirst for knowledge of the structure and function of the human body and a desire to apply that knowledge for the benefit of others who would become my patients. As the years passed, I had the good fortune of learning from many brilliant physicians and scientists. One such individual was Dr. Allan Pack at the University of Pennsylvania. Little did I know that Dr. Pack would become a world leader in the evolving science and practice of sleep medicine. In 1987, I had the privilege of joining the staff at Pennsylvania Hospital, the nation's first, founded by Benjamin Franklin in 1751.

While my primary focus was as a pulmonary and critical care medicine specialist, I came to the Pennsylvania Hospital with a newfound interest in obstructive sleep apnea syndrome. At Pennsylvania Hospital, I met Dr. Charles Cantor, a neurologist who shared my interest in sleep disorders. Together, in 1991, Dr. Cantor and I started a one-bed sleep center at Pennsylvania Hospital. As interest in sleep medicine grew in the community, so did requests for patient evaluations and sleep studies. Our program rapidly grew to a four-bed sleep center evaluating patients seven nights a week.

Through the years, Dr. Cantor has generously shared with me his knowledge and wisdom. Together we have evaluated and cared for thousands of patients with various sleep disorders. This book is a reflection of the collaborative effort Dr. Cantor and I have shared for over twenty years.

I wish to thank Dr. Alex Mason for his major contribution to this book in the area of children. Through his years of work in the field of pediatric sleep medicine, he has shared important insights regarding younger patients and their parents. I want to thank my highly skilled typist, Florence Nygaard, for her insights. I want to thank my medical partners, Dr. Michael Casey, Dr. Eugene Lugano, and Dr. Paul Kinniry. They have made me a better physician. I wish to acknowledge Dr. James Kearney of Otorhinolaryngology. Dr. Kearney is a talented surgeon who has provided excellent care for many of my patients through the years. He has also contributed valuable insights into the surgical management of snoring.

Lastly, I want to thank my coauthor, Maryann Karinch. She conceived the idea for this book and shared with us her extensive experience in writing multiple other great works on various subjects.

— *Ron Kotler*

Thanks to my mother, Ann, who taught me good sleep habits a long time ago. They seem to have stuck with me. Thank you to Jim for your moral support, patience and insights as I write, write, write. Thank you to my friends who always do what you can to help me rest well.

To my great partner in this adventure, Ron Kotler, who filled this project with intellectual energy and fun — thanks so much! And I very much appreciate the contributions of Charles Cantor, whose insights helped tremendously in this process, as well as Florence Nygaard, who helped get the manuscript in good order.

For the initial contributions to this work, I want to thank Ron Poropatich, an extraordinary physician and fine gentleman. I also send thanks to Jay Sanders for his keen medical insights, excellent guidance, and marvelous sense of humor. And to David Sherer—thanks for the reference! I've always known you to give great advice.

For tremendous support and guidance, I thank Meredith O'Hayre and Andrea Norville, our editors at Adams Media, where there is a publishing team I regard highly and enjoy every time we go around the block together. I also want to acknowledge Carolyn Wills and Tess Richardson for their wonderful guidance.

—Maryann Karinch

Foreword

Most of us take sleep for granted.

As individuals and as a species we have found ways to prolong our waking hours and to reduce the amount of time we spend asleep. For our ancestors, the relative length of the day and night was determined by the rotation of the earth. But we in the twenty-first century have uncoupled ourselves from this fundamental natural rhythm with artificial light, caffeine and medications, which allow us to manipulate our periods of sleep and wakefulness.

The result is that our need for sleep as an essential physiologic process has not been sufficiently acknowledged—by individuals, who may not be aware that they are sleep-deprived; by society, which places increasing demands upon our time in a shrinking world; and by the medical profession, which until recently has given insufficient attention to the role of sleep in promoting health.

This is beginning to change. Our understanding of sleep is expanding rapidly. At the same time as basic scientists are exploring the structure and functions of sleep, physicians are developing new insights into the mechanisms of sleep disorders and their treatment. We have learned, for example, that disturbances of breathing during sleep can have a significant impact on cardiovascular health, and that sleep deprivation can lead to profound impairment of work performance and intellectual function. We have developed new medications for narcolepsy, and new behavioral therapies for insomnia. We are investigating links between sleep and obesity and between sleep and longevity.

This book is designed to share this growing knowledge with you. It will help you educate yourself about sleep: what it is, why we need it, and how to achieve it.

You will find useful information here about both normal sleep and sleep disorders.

You will find guidance about how to handle a variety of sleep complaints, including excessive sleepiness, insomnia, and unusual behaviors that occur at night.

You will also find information about how sleep interacts with a number of medical conditions, and about how commonly used medications affect sleep.

You will learn how to identify sleep-related symptoms that require diagnosis and treatment by a sleep physician, and you will learn what an evaluation by a sleep physician involves.

The goal of the authors is to help you — regardless of your age and medical status — to understand and enjoy healthy sleep.

—Charles R. Cantor, MD, DABSM
Medical Director, Penn Sleep Centers

Introduction

Sleep has been demonstrated in mammals, birds, reptiles, and insects. The process we know as sleep is not unique to the human species. As necessary as it is, we still have questions about its role in human health and development. We know that babies sleep about 50 percent of the time, and as we get older, we sleep less and less. As we age, our sleep architecture changes such that less time is spent in deeper stages of sleep. Additionally, medical conditions and their treatments can have an adverse impact on sleep. There appear to be distinct relationships between changes in sleep and changes in brain development and function as we age. Many of these mysteries remain unsolved. Physicians and research scientists are working hard every day to enlighten us.

We know what we've observed: Sleep is important for memory, learning, and for feeling rested and well. Without an adequate amount of good sleep, we function at a sub optimal level and risk injury at work and while driving. If we repeatedly stop breathing during sleep, we risk premature death from heart attack or stroke.

When I was in medical school in the 1970s, the topic of sleep was ignored. We spend one third of our lives in this activity called sleep and I cannot remember a single lecture, much less an entire course, which touched on the subject.

The study of human sleep began to blossom in the 1950s with the development of EEG and the research published in 1953 by Eugene Aserinsky and Nathaniel Kleitman. Their work at the University of Chicago enabled identification of rapid eye movement sleep, the stage of sleep when we dream and experience skeletal muscle paralysis. They met a brilliant student named

William Dement, who later founded the world's first clinical sleep laboratory, located at Stanford University. His work led to the establishment of a medical specialty in sleep.

When I entered the specialty in the late 1980s, certified practitioners numbered fewer than 200. Now there are more than 1,000 accredited sleep centers and approximately 3,500 sleep specialists who have been certified by the American Board of Sleep Medicine. The invention of nasal CPAP by Colin E. Sullivan has given us the means to treat many patients who stop breathing during sleep. It has led to the explosive growth in interest in the field of sleep medicine. This simple device is dramatically effective in helping sufferers of the obstructive sleep apnea syndrome.

In this book, you will benefit from our journey as part of that growing group of specialists, as well as the body of knowledge that I personally have gained from over twenty years of clinical practice in aiding patients with sleep problems ranging from "Why can't I sleep?" to "Why am I so sleepy?"

If you have ever had trouble sleeping well, you have lots of company. Millions of people suffer from chronic problems that adversely affect sleep, such as obstructive sleep apnea, restless legs syndrome, and gastroesophageal reflux. At some point, we've all experienced insomnia, whether it was due to anxiety over a possible job loss, or the excitement of getting married. We will provide you with the tools to deal with the adverse impact that many of life's ups and downs will have on your nightly slumber. We believe that you will find something in this book to help you get a good night's sleep.

—Ronald Kotler, MD, DABSM
Medical Director, Pennsylvania Hospital Sleep Disorders Center

What You Need to Know about Sleep

The brain is normally in one of three physiologic states: awake, non–REM (rapid eye movement) sleep, or REM sleep. Unlike coma, sleep is a readily reversible state that will end when tactile stimulation or sound intervene, or when the cycle has simply run its course.

When and how much we sleep has two determinants: our sleep "debt," which accumulates as we spend time awake, and our circadian clock, located in the hypothalamus of the brain, which is normally linked to the twenty-four-hour light-dark cycle.

A complex sequence of activation and inhibition of different sites within the brain controls sleep and wakefulness. This sequence is highly organized, and as a result, different stages of sleep are apparent. As we become drowsy, we enter the lightest stage of sleep, referred to as Stage 1 sleep. We then descend into deeper sleep, passing through Stage 2 sleep until we arrive at slow-wave sleep, which is thought to be the stage that is essential for us to feel refreshed. We then ascend again into Stage 2 sleep, before entering rapid eye movement or REM sleep, which occurs about ninety to 120 minutes after we have fallen asleep. Adults typically cycle in and out of REM sleep every ninety to 120 minutes over the course of the night.

REM sleep is the stage of sleep in which we dream. REM has a number of other interesting characteristics as well:

- During REM sleep, our skeletal muscles are effectively paralyzed. The muscles that are spared include the diaphragm and the muscles controlling eye movements. Our arms and legs can twitch, but under normal circumstances they can't carry out prolonged or complex actions. This protects us from the injury that might occur if we were able to act out our dreams.

- Blood flow to the brain increases.
- Spontaneous erections in males and increased blood flow to the clitoris in females occur, unrelated to the content of dreams.
- Our heart rate and the rate and depth of breathing can fluctuate.
- Our ability to control body temperature is temporarily suspended.

Over our lifespan, the structure of sleep, or sleep architecture, changes. During the first year of life, the amount of time spent in REM sleep decreases from greater than half of total sleep time to about one third of total sleep time. In adulthood we spend about 20 to 25 percent of our time in REM sleep. As we age, the amount of slow-wave sleep decreases, and sleep in general is lighter, with more frequent arousals. Contrast this with a young child's sleep, which is so sound that you can move a napping child out of a car seat and into bed without waking him in the process. In the later stages of life, because we spend less time in deep sleep, we are more vulnerable to environmental disturbances, the effects of medications and the effects of medical conditions themselves.

Most adults, regardless of age, need seven to nine hours of sleep. If we are sleep-deprived, we are at risk of poor work performance, motor vehicle and industrial accidents, and disturbances of mood including depression and irritability. In addition, there is emerging evidence that poor sleep quality may be a factor in promoting obesity, diabetes, and in shortening life itself.

It is clear that to stay healthy and productive, good sleep is essential. Our goal in this book is to give you the tips and tools you need to achieve adequate and successful sleep.

1

advice for **everyone**

1. Aim for a Regular Schedule
2. Get 7½ to 8 Hours of Sleep
3. Allow Yourself Time to Prepare for Bed
4. Work in Synch with Your Own Circadian Rhythm
5. Take a Thirty-Minute Nap in the Afternoon
6. Avoid a Late-Afternoon Nap If You Have Insomnia
7. Don't Brood about Having a Bad Night
8. Associate Your Bedroom with Only Two Things
9. Get Out of Bed If You Can't Sleep
10. Take a Warm Bath
11. Wind Down at the End of the Day
12. Exercise Regularly
13. Get a Medical Checkup
14. Exercise No Later Than 3–4 Hours Before Bedtime
15. Let Nature Prepare You for Rest
16. Avoid Alcohol Before Bedtime
17. Avoid Caffeine Before Bedtime
18. Avoid Tobacco Before Bedtime

35. Don't Look at the Clock

36. Remind Your Friends and Family of Time Zones

37. Invest in a Decent Mattress

38. Don't Let Your Pet Sleep with You

39. Use Stress Management Techniques to Improve Sleep

40. Give Up the Mantra "If I Don't Have X Hours of Sleep, I Can't Function. . . ."

41. Calm Down from an Emotional High Before Bed

42. Save the Cough Drop for Daytime

43. Research Homeopathic Sleep Aids Before You Take Them

At some point, we've all had difficulty initiating and maintaining sleep, which is how sleep doctors characterize "insomnia." Good sleep hygiene refers to healthful practices that help you fall asleep and maintain restful sleep. Whether or not you have any difficulty sleeping, these tips apply.

Some of the tips in Chapter 10: Advice on Alternative Therapies also relate to strategies that have a general, positive effect on your sleep experience, such as yoga stretches before bedtime. The tips in this chapter fall into the category of advice physicians will commonly give when a person has trouble sleeping. The tips in Chapter 10 come from professionals in fields such as physical therapy, homeopathy, and massage.

1. Aim for a Regular Schedule

When you go to bed and get out of bed at the same time every day, you greatly increase your chances of getting restful sleep. Even if you have to deviate from your routine a couple of nights a week because of work, classes, kids' schedules, or volunteer activities, do whatever you can to avoid extreme changes in your sleep schedule. Significant deviations from your normal pattern can throw your system off and lead to sleep disruption. Weekend partying is a classic example of how you can disturb your sleep cycle. If you stay up late on Saturday night and then sleep until noon on Sunday, you may have trouble falling asleep at a reasonable hour on Sunday night. That means you will start the week short on sleep. Frequent variations in your schedule will undermine the brain's ability to maintain a regular pattern of sleep and wakefulness, leading to difficulties in falling asleep, waking up, and remaining alert at appropriate times.

2. Get 7½ to 8 Hours of Sleep

Realistically, you will sometimes face situations with travel, meetings, and other demands that keep you from getting adequate sleep. But do what you can to get it—and that doesn't mean just lying in bed for 7½ to 8 hours. It means using the tips in this book to make sure you actually sleep that amount of time.

3. Allow Yourself Time to Prepare for Bed

Scheduling for the right amount of sleep means allowing yourself time to prepare for sleep. Your bedtime ritual may include a number of activities: locking up, checking on children, bathing, flossing, and so on. Remember that this does not count as sleep time.

4. Work in Synch with Your Own Circadian Rhythm

Circadian rhythm (Latin: circa = around; dies = day) roughly means a twenty-four-hour cycle. It refers to the biorhythms of the brain. Circadian rhythms control a number of familiar functions, such as sleep, appetite, and blood levels of certain hormones according to a daily pattern. Our circadian rhythm tells us that we should be awake about sixteen hours and asleep about eight hours. The sleep-wake cycle of twenty-four hours, therefore, reflects the fact that we "allow" ourselves to adjust to a rhythm that corresponds to a single day. Light serves as an important cue to the part of the brain known as the hypothalamus to keep us in synch with the day-night cycle related to the rotating earth. A normal part of the circadian rhythm for wakefulness is that it takes a dip in the afternoon—and the timing and level of that dip can differ from person to person. So it's normal to feel a little sluggish around the time that a lot of people in San Juan and Madrid take a siesta; these cultures have recognized that Mother Nature has made us sleepier in the mid-afternoon. The business executive who takes off at 3:00 P.M. and goes to the gym to work out is using exercise rather than napping to cope with the mid-afternoon circadian dip. Lifting weights and running on a treadmill require no particular mental invest-ment. On the other hand, reading a technical paper with the hope of presenting it at a meeting the next day is something you would be better off doing at 10:00 A.M. than 3:00 P.M. If you pay attention to your circadian rhythm, then you will ease into a sleep-wake cycle that is normal for you.

5. Take a Thirty-Minute Nap in the Afternoon

For those who feel a lull and have the luxury of taking a siesta (or power nap, depending on where you're from), that's fine. It reflects the dip in circadian rhythm that is normal for human beings. The potential danger of napping is taking too many naps in a day, napping for too long or too late in the day. Naps are also a risk for those who have insomnia, as explained in the next tip.

6. Avoid a Late-Afternoon Nap If You Have Insomnia

If you like to nap, stick to mid-afternoon. Don't sprawl on the couch at 6:00 P.M. and fall asleep as you wait for someone to call you to the dinner table. If you have trouble falling asleep or staying asleep at night, keep in mind that any daytime sleep may lessen your drive to sleep at night.

7. Don't Brood about Having a Bad Night

While you need a good night's sleep to function at your peak, missing a few hours of sleep one night will not necessarily ruin your day. Have an extra cup of coffee, get on with your life, and get the sleep you need the next night. Don't let your concern for an occasional bad night of sleep spiral out of control into an obsession. There is a specific cognitive distortion called the fortune-telling error, in which you predict that bad things will happen even though you have no good evidence that they will. This type of distorted thinking is described by Dr. David D. Burns in his book *Feeling Good, the New Mood Therapy*. Confront this cognitive distortion by recognizing it for what it is—an exaggeration. Substitute the thought for a more realistic one: Everyone from time to time has a bad night; that doesn't mean every night will be bad. Don't let your fear and anxiety about sleep become a self-fulfilling prophecy.

8. Associate Your Bedroom with Only Two Things

You need to train your brain to link the bedroom with sleep and relaxing pleasure. The bed should therefore be reserved for sleep and sexual activity. You can develop "psycho-physiologic insomnia" by repeatedly doing things in the bedroom that run counter to sleep. This is similar to the conditioned reflex-reaction that Pavlov's dogs had in response to hearing a bell: He trained them to associate the bell with eating, so that even when the bell didn't lead to dinner, the dogs still salivated. So if going to bed to you means watching raucous reruns of Miami Vice while munching on potato chips, then you are not conditioning yourself to associate the bed with sleep. Maybe you're the ambitious type who takes your Blackberry or iPhone to bed to do one last e-mail check before sleeping, or make a few notes about the next day's meetings. That's just as bad. You need to look at the bed and feel as though it represents a vacation; you should feel happy to be there. Condition yourself to see the bed as the place for good quality sleep.

9. Get Out of Bed If You Can't Sleep

You condition yourself to associate insomnia with the bed by allowing yourself to lie awake tossing and turning for hours. Your brain starts to see the bed as a place for worry and unrest. If you find yourself struggling to sleep for half an hour or more (or if it feels like half an hour or more), then move to a different room. Sit quietly in a dimly lit room and read something monotonous until you feel like sleeping. This is one way of adjusting your surroundings to create a more desirable stimulus-response relationship.

10. Take a Warm Bath

Immersing yourself in a warm bath before bedtime can be very relaxing and very soothing. It can help relieve aching muscles and tension that may interfere with sleep onset. Try using bath oil with lavender in it; the aroma has been known to relax and aid in sleep.

11. Wind Down at the End of the Day

Having a period of winding down as you get to the end of your day helps your brain shift gradually to a lower gear. Give yourself a couple of hours to move into a state of relaxation. Give in completely to the need to unwind; get your body and your brain in the mood to sleep.

12. Exercise Regularly

Aerobic exercise has many benefits. It can improve cardiovascular health. It can promote weight loss, and it can provide a sense of well-being. Maintaining a normal weight helps to avoid arthritic pain, reflux, and disturbances of breathing during sleep. The reduction in stress and the elevation in mood, which can result from regular exercise, can help consolidate sleep.

13. Get a Medical Checkup

Prior to entering into a vigorous aerobic exercise program to aid your sleep and overall health, check with your physician. If you have been sedentary for many years, you will want to make sure your heart can handle the increased workload of strenuous activity. Any personal trainer certified by organizations such as the American Council on Exercise (ACE) or National Strength and Conditioning

Association has learned the protocols that relate to screening and will ask you for your physician's written okay to proceed if you have a pre-existing medical condition. ACE also provides courses enabling certified trainers to earn their credentials as certified exercise specialists who know how to work with special populations such as people with heart disease, fibromyalgia, and a host of other medical conditions that interrupt sleep. If you have a concern, ask if the trainers at your gym have these credentials.

14. Exercise No Later Than 3–4 Hours Before Bedtime

Vigorous exercise causes the release of hormones and changes in body tempera-ture that may make it more difficult to fall asleep. One of the hormones released is adrenaline, that "fight or flight" juice that puts your body in a high-energy state. Vigorous exercise may stimulate your brain and muscles at a time when you should be relaxed. In contrast, gentle stretching or walking are types of exercise that can be helpful to sleep, and specific ways to do it are addressed in Chapter 10.

15. Let Nature Prepare You for Rest

Sit outside after dinner, or take a stroll, ideally with someone you can talk with. The gentle exercise of a slow walk has value in the early evening a couple of hours before bedtime

16. Avoid Alcohol Before Bedtime

Feet on the ottoman, you watch Conan O'Brien's monologue as you finish your second glass of wine. The relaxing sensation kicks in by the first commercial and you shuffle off to bed. You wake up three hours later, shifting under the covers and thirsty. Alcohol is a terrible "nightcap": Drinking before bedtime can lead to the onset of sleep because it is sedating, but it results in fragmented sleep for people with no health issues and exacerbates sleep problems for people who snore or stop breathing. As the body withdraws from the alcohol, the brain gets excited. Sleep becomes lighter. Whether you have insomnia or not, alcohol is not something you want in your system as you drive toward dreamland.

17. Avoid Caffeine Before Bedtime

Unlike alcohol, caffeine is a stimulant—and a powerful one for many people. If you have the double whammy of reacting acutely to caffeine and not sleeping well, avoid caffeine for twelve hours before bedtime. Don't just pass on the after-dinner coffee. Pass on the lunchtime cola and mid-morning coffee, too. The fact is, caffeine can stay in your body for fourteen hours, so sensitivity to it could mean that you have to stop ingesting coffee, teas, soda, and chocolate fourteen hours before you intend to go to bed. Be sure to read labels. The soda you ingest may contain caffeine.

18. Avoid Tobacco Before Bedtime

We know that smoking is bad for sleep since nicotine, which is found in tobacco products, is a stimulant. Knowing the long-term effects of smoking on lung function, we also believe there may be a respiratory component to the effect on sleep as well. A combined team of researchers from the Complutense School of Medicine in Madrid and UCLA School of Medicine in Los Angeles decided to look closely at that assumption to document the effects of smoking on respiratory activity during sleep. They found that, among this group of "healthy" smokers, smoking did decrease the amount of oxygen they were able to take in during sleep. We can speculate that, although the people who participated in the study are healthy now, they may be courting medical problems.

19. Drink Warm Herbal Tea

Chamomile or other herbal teas may have a calming effect as your body takes in the warmth of hot tea (without caffeine). Sit back and relax. Enjoy the soothing moment. Forget about the stresses from earlier in the day.

20. Don't Watch TV in Bed

Hotels set you up for sleep failure with the television just beyond the foot of the bed and a remote on the bed stand. Don't make the same mistake in your own home. Your bed has been designed for sleep, regardless of what you might think. Allow it to function properly by keeping your eyes off the TV whenever you want to sleep. TV works against sleep in several ways. You might delay sleeping until a show is over. If you do fall asleep, you could be disturbed by sudden loud noises or waking up to turn off the tube. Another unhappy outcome: You fall asleep only to incorporate a cast of bad characters in your nightmare. In addition to the possibility of unexpected noises, absorbing plot twists, and shocking images, the most fundamental reason you should not watch TV in bed is that the bright light stimulates you. Light helps to regulate your sleep-wake cycle; exposing yourself to light has an arousal effect. Light exposure can fool your brain into thinking it is time to be awake and alert.

21. Abandon Your Gadgets

Unless you're playing a boring podcast or easy listening music, your electronic gadgets have no place in or near the bed. One exception is the phone next to your bed. Use it only for emergencies. You never know when a conversation in the bedroom will lead to feelings of excitement, guilt, or anxiety. These emotions are not conducive to sleep. Use a phone in another room for daily chatting.

22. Move the Computer

Keep your computer outside of the bedroom. Late night e-mails, games, and instant messaging will cut into sleep time. Finish your work and your play on the computer well before bedtime and don't give yourself easy access to your computer by putting it in the same room as your bed. Out of sight, out of mind.

23. Choose Light Bedtime Reading

Reading at bedtime is a good way to drift off to sleep, however don't choose anything that will provoke strong thoughts or emotions. If you're a magazine reader rather than book reader, choose your articles well. Go with the movie review and pop culture chapters of the news magazines instead of reading about the failing economy or urban violence. Reading an exciting or absorbing book can be fine as long as the content isn't upsetting or so thought provoking that your mind leaps into action.

24. Make a List of Things That Help You Sleep

When going to sleep, the brain attempts to block out stimuli, and when the brain isn't successful, it needs a little help. What are the things that you think help you relax? Different people have different arousal thresholds. A young child has a very high arousal threshold during sleep, to the point where you can pick him up out of the car and transfer him to the bed without waking him up. As we get older, we awaken more easily due to external stimuli. Every individual has to define personally what kind of environment and bedtime activities are conducive to sleep. If you want to sleep with a teddy bear because it helps you relax, then do it.

25. Block Out Stimuli

An eye mask and earplugs can cut down on the disruption from streetlights and the sounds of cars, or if you live in the mountains, the light of a really bright moon and the howling winds.

26. Replace Stimuli with Soothing Sounds

Supposedly, the great comedian W.C. Fields needed the sound of rain on the roof to get a restful sleep. Some people rely on devices that recreate the sound of the ocean. We have friends living near a bay who realized, when they couldn't get to sleep one night that it was because the sound of the foghorn had ceased. Some upstart new neighbors had complained about it and the port authorities responded by turning it off. So many people complained about not having the foghorn sound at night, however, that the decision was quickly reversed.

27. Recreate a Soothing Atmosphere While Away from Home

Find a way to make sights and sounds the same. Just like the people who wanted the foghorn at night, you may find that traveling or moving to a new home will present you with differences in stimuli that make sleeping difficult. Try to remember what worked for you previously, and then to whatever extent possible, recreate the atmosphere.

28. Pay Your Sleep Debts

After a work- or school-week of getting five hours of sleep a night, you should try to catch up. Most people don't want to give up their weekends to sleep, but it's important to find at least a few more hours of sleep to avoid problems associated with sleep deprivation. The drive for sleep increases as you are up longer and longer. When you get up in the morning and you haven't slept well, you are still relatively alert because your circadian drive for wakefulness is strong. When you will really crash is when your circadian rhythm is at its low point and, at the same time, your sleepiness is at a high point. That happens at bedtime primarily and to a lesser extent in the afternoon. If you are not getting seven to nine hours of sleep each night as we recommend, you will be particularly sleepy in the afternoon and evening and your performance is likely to be impaired throughout the day.

29. Avoid a Big Meal Before Bed

Eating too close to bedtime means your body is busy digesting instead of winding down for a long rest. Digestion involves corrosive stomach acids, so you have the added possibility that you will get indigestion because you are lying down while the process of breaking down food is going on. When you fill your stomach with food, remain in a sitting or standing position for several hours afterwards. Gravity helps move the food into your intestines. Trying to digest while in a supine position takes gravity out of the equation; that cheese steak just sits there in your stomach, or worse yet, moves up into your esophagus and even your lungs. The burning sensation of the corrosive acids in your esophagus is called reflux. Hoarseness and impaired breathing can result, but so can far worse problems. We've seen patients come in for emergency care because they woke up suddenly with a high fever and cough caused by pneumonia induced by late night eating. Food and acid came up into the esophagus, went through the vocal cords, and then descended into the lungs. Eating late at night can cause weight gain, and make your sleep restless, but it can have more serious implications as well.

30. Start Your Sleep in a Chair If You Ate a Big Meal

On those rare occasions when eating a meal occurs late, start your sleep in a chair. Dim the lights, put your feet on the ottoman and snooze for a few hours in your La-Z-Boy after coming home from the party.

31. Eat a Light Snack Before Bed

If you like to use food as part of a self-soothing ritual, eat a light snack. While a big meal can cause problems at bedtime, a little late-night snack can serve you. Some people have a little bowl of cereal when they don't feel sleepy at bedtime, and others like a piece of toast and low-acid fruit. Carbohydrates seem to promote sleepiness more than other types of foods. Some people get the same response from a cup of soup. The trick is to keep the amount small and the food relatively light.

32. Complete Preparations for the Next Day Before Going to Bed

Help take your mind off planning details in bed by attending to those details earlier, in a room other than the bedroom.

33. Empty Your Mind of Disruptive Thoughts

If the to-dos still pile up and wake you up after you've gone to bed, then get up and make a list. Sit quietly and write down all of the items that pull your brain out of sleep and then look at them logically. You can't attend that big meeting right now. You can't call the plumber right now. You can't pick your kid up from school right now. You have your list and you can see for yourself that all you can actually do now is go to sleep and deal with it the next day. With this exercise, you literally and symbolically empty your mind of disruptive thoughts.

34. Steer Yourself Away from Troublesome Thoughts by Focusing on the Inconsequential

Traditionally, this occurs by counting sheep. You can also try to remember every phone number you ever had, all the presidents of the United States, or everybody in your Facebook file. You begin to create a list that means absolutely nothing and fall asleep before it ever takes shape. Perhaps this is effective because it distracts you from more emotionally charged thoughts that keep you awake.

35. Don't Look at the Clock

If you wake up in the middle of the night, don't look at the clock. Sounds trivial, but this can have a significant impact on your ability to go back to sleep. Looking at the clock tends to generate worry and calculations: "If I don't fall asleep within the next fifteen minutes, then I will not get the amount I need to feel good tomorrow. That will ruin my presentation. I'll get fired from my job..." Set an alarm you trust will awaken you in the morning and then turn the clock around or put it under the bed where it is out of sight.

36. Remind Your Friends and Family of Time Zones

If you live on the West coast, remind your family and friends on the East coast of the three-hour difference. You won't want them calling you at 8:00 A.M. their time because that just might interrupt your sleep. Conversely, if you live on the East coast, remind your friends and family on the West coast that your time zone is three hours later. You won't want them calling you from a party at 10:00 P.M. to say, "Hi."

37. Invest in a Decent Mattress

How many of us have parents who still sentimentally sleep (or try to) on the mattress they had when they were first wed? When a mattress has lumps, tears, sags, or smells, get rid of it. The Better Sleep Council (*www.bettersleep.org*) describes a decent "Sleep Test" as the following:

- Select a mattress
- Lie down in your sleep position
- Evaluate the level of comfort and support
- Educate yourself about each selection
- Partners should try each mattress together

Dr. Clete A. Kushida, a spokesman for the American Academy of Sleep Medicine and the director of the Stanford Center for Human Sleep Research at Stanford University concurs with the test-drive approach. He says, "Lie on your side. If your shoulders and hips are sinking, if you feel your spine is not aligned, it's probably too soft. If you feel pain and discomfort, it's probably too firm" (*www.webmd.com*). Make sure the mattress you buy has a thirty-day money back guarantee because you really won't know whether it's the right mattress for you until you sleep on it.

38. Don't Let Your Pet Sleep with You

To get a good night's sleep, you'll need to train your pets to sleep in their own beds. Many people have no problem saying "sleep in your own bed" to their restless child, but when it comes to droop-eared, sad-eyed Sparky, they cave in. Unless you have a large bed, sleep alone, and Sparky stays in one spot all night, do yourself and your bed partner a favor and send Sparky to his own bed. Same for cute little Fluffy. Not only can dogs and cats make space and attention demands that disrupt sleep, but they can also leave behind hair and dander that cause respiratory problems related to allergies and asthma. It's not cruel to give them their own special beds—really.

39. Use Stress Management Techniques to Improve Sleep

Worry is the enemy of sleep. Although it is virtually impossible for you to avoid stress in your life, it is important to have a strategy for dealing with worries before they begin to dominate your thoughts. This is a particular risk at night, when there are few distractions. Poor sleep results. A number of stress management and relaxation techniques have been developed to help people cope with both transient and long-term concerns. Cognitive behavioral therapy (CBT) can be particularly helpful when anxiety disrupts your sleep. Developed to treat mood disorders, including depression and anxiety, CBT enables people to recognize and avoid patterns of thought that, at best, are unproductive and, at worst, distort reality. A specific form of CBT has been developed to treat insomnia. Many psychiatrists, psychologists and other trained counselors—often affiliated with a sleep center—have expertise in the use of CBT. For many people with insomnia, CBT is an effective alternative to the use of sleeping pills.

40. Give Up the Mantra "If I Don't Have X Hours of Sleep, I Can't Function. . . ."

One of the most pernicious obsessions people can have related to sleep is to assume that they require a specific amount of sleep each night in order to function at all. We have seen cases where the obsession with a specific quantity of sleep becomes so persistent that the patient's thinking becomes almost psychotic. Such patients may need care from a psychiatrist. In less severe cases, the focus on relatively mild sleep deprivation can lead to a self-fulfilling prophecy: It is actually the worry about inadequate sleep that is keeping the patient awake. If you need a mantra, use a more sensible one: "If I get any sleep, I'm ready for action."

41. Calm Down from an Emotional High Before Bed

Remember the night before school started? The night before your wedding? Clearly, it isn't just trauma that gives you acute insomnia (unless you consider school or weddings traumatic). You need to take extra pre-sleep steps to counter the effects of extreme anticipation, just as you do if you're distressed. In addition to those hot baths and glasses of warm milk, in the days before the event, take walks and let your mind envision the details of your concert, or wedding, or speech as you get some exercise. When other people say, "What can I do to help?" be prepared with answers that take pressure off you to "fix" things. Have checklists ready for your helpers. Make plans for important events during the daytime so that your mind can turn to more relaxing thoughts at night.

42. Save the Cough Drop for Daytime

Post-nasal drip is a common cause of cough that can suddenly interfere with sleep, but there are ways to mitigate the problem without falling asleep with a cough drop in your mouth and running the risk of needing a Heimlich maneuver. To eliminate post-nasal drip, identify the cause. Some people have seasonal or situational allergies, which cause allergic rhinitis. Vasomotor rhinitis (VMR) is the non-allergic type, which may be triggered by something controllable like cigarette smoke in your house, or uncontrollable like a sudden change in barometric pressure or temperature. In both cases, fluids collect in back of your airway and a cough results. Treatment of vasomotor rhinitis should start with avoiding conditions that you know will cause it. When this fails, or when precipitating factors are unavoidable, nasal sprays may be beneficial. These include an anti-inflammatory nasal steroid or an anticholinergic spray known as ipratropium bromide. While oral decongestants may also prove beneficial, they can be stimulating and contribute to sleep disruption. If you have a chronic issue, ask your doctor to advise you. But save the tongue-numbing, cherry-flavored lumps for daytime.

43. Research Homeopathic Sleep Aids Before You Take Them

Always do your research before taking "natural" sleep aids. Put your focus on assessing the quality control measures that the manufacturer takes, and knowing exactly what dosage is recommended for your body weight, gender, and age. The hormone melatonin, for example, is secreted by the body naturally, but the doses that should be used as a supplement are not clearly established, nor is the drug regulated by the Food and Drug Administration. In terms of dosage, you don't really know how much would benefit you, because your weight and natural melatonin production are key factors that determine response. The usual dosages range from 3 to 6 mg.

2

Advice for People Who Sleep **Too Little**

96. Check for Bacterial Infection and Parasites

97. Get Enough Sleep Before You Drive

98. Know the Signs of Drowsy Driving

99. Get a Room

100. Late at Night, You Should Be Sleeping, Not Driving

101. Make Sure Your Teen Gets Enough Sleep Before Handing Over the Keys

102. Tell Your Parents You're Concerned about Their Driving If They Have Sleep Problems

103. If You Drive a Bus or Truck, Society Depends on You to Be Alert

104. If You Work Twenty-Four Hours Straight, Sleep When You Get Home and Not While You're Driving

105. Close Your Window During Allergy Season

106. Don't Overuse Over-the-Counter Nasal Sprays

107. Get a Prescription Nasal Spray

108. Block Out Dust Mites

109. Lose the Feather Pillow

110. Invest in an Air Filter

Some people deal with a life-long difficulty in falling asleep or remaining asleep, regardless of their circumstances. There is some evidence that such people have naturally fragile sleep with frequent arousals and sensitivity to environmental disturbances. If the sleep tips in Chapter 1 were not enough to help you, then let this guidance take you a little deeper into the issues and answers.

Some of the specific difficulties covered here involve:

- Relationship incompatibilities
- Traveling
- Allergies

The presence of any of these does not indicate you have a sleep disorder, but they may be the cause of your sleeping too little.

44. Don't Assume You've Lost Your Ability to Sleep

People who label themselves insomniacs often deal with a problem called sleep state misperception, which means they are actually getting much more sleep than they think. We can document this during sleep studies by asking the patients, "How much sleep did you get last night?" They tell us they hardly slept at all, or estimate that it was maybe an hour, but we know that they slept for several hours. So if your gauge of whether or not you have had restful sleep is simply how many hours you believe you slept, it's time to stop looking at the clock and start focusing more on your level of daytime functioning. Sleepiness can be assessed with the Epworth Sleepiness Scale. Get your Epworth Sleepiness Scale score by turning to Appendix A and taking the test.

45. Spend Less Time in Bed

Lying awake in bed is not productive; in fact it generally increases performance anxiety about sleep. If you have trouble falling asleep, you shouldn't go to bed until you are very sleepy. This principle underlies a more complex insomnia treatment known as sleep restriction. Patients being treated with sleep restriction are instructed to go to bed much later than their desired bedtime. This helps to change their focus from "How can I fall asleep at bedtime?" to "How can I stay awake as late as my sleep physician recommended?" By the time you are allowed to go to bed, you will most likely be so tired that you will fall asleep more easily than usual. Once you are able to consistently fall asleep quickly at the new bedtime, you should be able to cautiously advance your bedtime to an earlier hour, under the direction of a sleep physician or cognitive behavioral therapist.

46. Try a Mild Sleep Aid

When sleep-hygiene measures aren't quite enough, try a mild sleep aid. Modern medicine has developed some effective, non-addictive drugs to aid sleep. They have quick onset of action and, generally speaking, no hangover or major residual effects as long as you allow yourself a full eight hours of sleep after you take them. They are not intended to be a lifelong aid, though. During menopause, after the death of a loved one, and under a number of other disrupting circumstances faced by otherwise normal, healthy people, the temporary use of sleeping pills is often okay. "If they're so benign, then why not use them all the time?" you ask. Even really "good" drugs have potential side effects. Users of sleeping pills need to be wary of a number of potential side effects including residual sedation that can impair coordination, thinking or behavior. This is a particular risk in the elderly. Psychological dependence on sleeping pills and tolerance of a given dose can develop in the absence of true physical addiction. And if you're already a snorer, then taking sleeping pills could exacerbate that problem. All decisions about the long-term use of sleep medications should be made on a case-by-case basis with your physician, taking into account age, regular alcohol use, which would preclude the use of sleeping medications, prior history of drug or medication dependence, and job requirements, which may be incompatible with the use of sedating drugs.

47. Use Other Types of Medication to Help You Sleep

It may be okay to use drugs not designed as sleeping pills to help you sleep. As long as the suggestion comes from your doctor, you may be able to use certain antidepressants, muscle relaxants and antihistamines to help you sleep. Sometimes long-term use of these drugs can be helpful to patients who have a chronic medical problem, for example depression or pain, in addition to insomnia. Refer to Appendix B for a table of common medications.

48. Do Not Use Stimulants as a Substitute for Sleep

Stimulants do not replace sleep, which is an essential biologic function. In our society, you can obtain stimulants in a variety of ways and many forms; use them all with caution. Prescribed stimulants should be used only as directed, and not to keep you going when you need rest. They have a significant abuse potential. Even caffeine causes side effects when used to excess.

49. Ask Yourself If You're a Night Owl

Delayed Sleep Phase can masquerade as primary insomnia. If you have always been a "night owl" who has had trouble falling asleep until after midnight, you may have a delayed sleep phase. The hallmark of this condition is that you do not become sleepy until the early morning hours and your natural tendency is to sleep late into the late morning or early afternoon. This is a common occurrence in adolescence. If you go to bed late but are able to sleep until you wake up naturally, feeling refreshed, then you need not worry. But a delayed sleep phase is often incompatible with the demands of school or work, and there are ways to re-align your sleep pattern with correctly timed exposure to bright light. This condition is discussed further in Chapter 4: Advice for People Who Sleep at the Wrong Time.

50. Find Out If You're Truly a "Short Sleeper"

You can mask a physiologic tendency toward sleepiness by staying active. We see a lot of patients who think nothing is seriously wrong because they can manage to stay awake despite the short amount of time they devote to sleep: "I'm fine as long as I'm moving," they say. Many of these people seek out a physician, not because they feel particularly tired, but because they have a spouse who complains about their bedtime behavior: snoring, cessation of breathing while sleeping, teeth grinding, sleepwalking, and so on. It's normal for a lot of people to feel sluggish when they first get up, and then feel fine the rest of the day. It's not normal to feel awake only when you're active. Studies have shown that people can fool themselves into thinking they have achieved peak, or nearly peak, performance in a sleep deprived state, but that self-assessment is way off. They are completely unaware of the fact that there is a marked difference between how they do a task after refreshing sleep and how they handle it when they aren't rested. There is a subset of the human population that just doesn't need the same amount of sleep, but these "short sleepers" are rare. A true short sleeper will consistently feel well rested, even with inactivity, after less than six hours of nightly sleep.

51. Avoid Stimulating Medications Before Bed

Some prescription and over-the-counter medications are either designed to wake you up or have stimulation as a side effect. The most common one used to be the decongestant pseudoephedrine, but its role in making "crystal meth" caused some manufacturers to remove it from their cold remedies. Asthma inhalers are another common culprit. Check the fine print on all drugs you take and, if one of the side effects is listed as "agitation" or "stimulation," then let it wear off well before bedtime. But be sure to speak to your health care provider before changing or discontinuing any prescribed medication.

52. Sleep in a Quieter, Darker Environment

Get a quieter, darker environment if you're having more sleep challenges as you age. As you age, you will experience a decrease in slow-wave sleep. This leads to lighter sleep and greater susceptibility to noise, ambient temperature changes, pain, and discomfort. Alter your sleeping quarters to whatever extent you can to accommodate your new needs.

53. Mute Your Pain Before Bed

Whether mild or severe, pain can disrupt sleep. Not all types of pain require medication, however. A headache resulting from stress might go away quickly with a massage. Pain related to an old sports injury, for example, may only occur when your body is in a particular position, so take precautions (like piling pillows) to stay out of that position. For many types of pain, though, the right dose of medication for pain relief—no more, no less—will give you important hours of restful sleep. Take it at least thirty minutes before going to bed so that it kicks in before you slip under the covers. You want to associate the bed with comfort and sleep, not the fight against pain. If your medical regimen does not consistently provide adequate pain relief, talk to your health care provider.

54. Avoid Nasal Dryness

Use a saline nasal spray if you live in or visit a dry climate. Nasal congestion, and even nasal bleeding, can result from exposure to dry climates and can contribute to sleep disruption. Use an over-the-counter saline nasal spray right before you go to bed to minimize the effect of the dryness.

55. Invest in a Humidifier

If you live in a dry climate, a humidifier can be a big help. The soothing effects of a saline nasal spray may not be enough, depending on where you live. Humidifiers can be very quiet and suitable for the bedroom, so if you frequently wake up with discomfort due to the dryness, invest in a small, portable humidifier.

56. Visit Your Doctor If You Have Night Sweats

With the onset of night sweats, go to the doctor. Excessive sweating in bed to the point where you have to change your pajamas or sheets should not happen when you sleep. You get relief from a normal sweat by kicking off the covers or lowering the temperature in the room. But you will get no relief, even when you take those actions, if your sweating is due to a medical problem. The range of such problems runs from annoying, but predictable—for example, menopause—to potentially life-threatening. Some menopausal women choose to get some rest with the help of a light sleeping pill. For others, estrogen replacement therapy can work well; still others find relief with black cohosh, an herb used in Native American medicine. (Also see Chapter 10: Advice on Alternative Therapies.) Other causes of night sweats can be more serious: obstructive sleep apnea, reflux, systemic infections like tuberculosis, and thyroid problems.

57. Wear Light Clothing to Bed
Some menopausal women lose hours of sleep night after night due to hot flashes. You can try sleeping in very light clothes; some manufacturers offer PJs in special "dry" fabrics for people who suffer from night sweats.

58. Use a Fan
Cool down with the help of a fan. Some women find relief for their menopausal night sweats in air blowing gently over them. Position a fan so you can feel the breeze, but don't use one of those moving fans or your partner may find a reason to pull the plug on it.

59. Avoid Spicy Foods
Avoid spicy foods if you're prone to night sweats. Hot peppers can make you hot—literally.

60. Get Checked for Diabetes

If you have frequent episodes of urination at night, ask your doctor to check you for diabetes. Nocturnal urination can be caused by an enlarged prostate in men, by obstructive sleep apnea, and by diabetes. Diabetes is characterized by a deficiency in insulin production. This leads to an increase of sugar in your blood. When the increased sugar circulates through the kidneys, it causes an increase in urine output. Frequent nocturnal awakenings due to a need to urinate may be a sign that you have developed diabetes. Other symptoms include increased thirst and increased hunger. Diabetes is the number one cause of blindness in the United States. Additionally, it can cause kidney failure requiring dialysis, and heart attacks. It also increases the risk of neurologic problems including stroke, nerve damage, and impaired emptying of the stomach. If you are an adult onset diabetic, there is a good chance that you also have obstructive sleep apnea. Treating your apnea may help you to control your blood sugar.

RELATIONSHIP INCOMPATIBILITIES

61. Designate a Time for Cuddling

Have designated "cuddle time"—and then agree with your partner on when to end it—if the proximity keeps you awake. You can love someone deeply, find him (or her) exceedingly sexy, and just not want to cuddle. Make it clear to a partner who wants to spoon 'til dawn that you need to limit your cuddle time or risk falling asleep at the wheel.

62. Resolve Thermal Incompatibility

Couples commonly have different temperature needs for a comfortable sleep, so the objective is to find a way to give you both what you want all the time. If one likes windows open for cold air, or air conditioning that could freeze a steak, then the one who needs warmth must have the option of blankets. Often, an electric blanket with dual controls is the best answer. One side can be completely off while the other can be on high and, as long as no one violates the terms of the cuddling arrangement, you should be able to achieve thermal compatibility.

63. Establish Compatible Sleep Rituals

For two people who are rigid and uncompromising about their sleep needs—for example, one must watch television, but the other must read in silence—sleep becomes the focal point for underlying relationship difficulties. Focus on what those difficulties are and, if you can resolve them, then you are on the way to eliminating the problems related to sleep. If you can't resolve them, then you will still be able to get rid of your sleep problems—by sleeping alone.

64. Don't Think Separate Beds Means a Bad Relationship

A lot of new homes are being built with two master bedrooms to accommodate people who want to stay together, but sleep better apart. For people with totally incompatible sleep schedules and habits, that may be the only way to stay together.

TRAVELING

65. Beware of Jet Lag

When you travel, you create a circadian rhythm disorder for yourself if you cross multiple time zones. You may have no sleeping problems at home, but when you arrive on foreign soil, your body clock is suddenly hours behind (or ahead) of local time. Depending on the distance and direction you have traveled, jet lag can cause sleepiness, insomnia, and gastrointestinal symptoms. The good news is that exposure to the light-dark cycle in your new time zone will eventually reset your body clock to local time. Recommendations for the quickest adjustment of your body clock are summarized below.

66. Fly at a Time That Puts You in Synch with Your Destination Time Zone as Soon as Possible

If you are flying from the West coast of the United States to the East coast, for example, leave very early in the morning so that you are tired when it's bedtime on the East coast.

67. When Flying East, Seek Sunlight in the Morning

If you are crossing up to six time zones and flying east, seek exposure to sunlight in the morning. Since your circadian rhythm at home is delayed (your bedtime is later) relative to your destination, you need early morning light exposure, as you would in the treatment of a delayed sleep phase.

68. When Flying West, Seek Sunlight in the Evening

If you are crossing up to six time zones flying west, seek exposure to sunlight in the evening. Since your circadian rhythm at home is advanced (your bedtime is earlier) relative to your destination, you need evening light exposure, as you would in the treatment of an advanced sleep phase.

69. If You Are Crossing More Than Six Time Zones, You Will Need to Make a More Complicated Adjustment

In this case, the timing of light exposure upon arrival may be confusing to the body clock, which may mistake early morning light for evening light or vice versa. When crossing more than six time zones flying east, you should not seek morning light exposure until several days have passed, to minimize the risk of further delaying your sleep phase. Similarly, when crossing more than six time zones flying west, you should not seek evening light exposure for several days to minimize the risk of further advancing your sleep phase.

70. Use Medication to Sleep While Traveling

Consider the use of hypnotic medications to help you sleep while flying or to help overcome insomnia while becoming adjusted to local time. Discuss the temporary use of sleeping pills to help counteract jet lag with your doctor.

71. Don't Sleep Continuously on a Long Flight

If you're at risk for blood clots, don't sleep continuously on the airplane. Unless you have the luxury of getting your own bed to stretch out on your next transatlantic flight, you will likely be cramped into a small seat with little room to move for a pro-longed period of time. While you will be tempted to take a sleeping pill so you can wake up in Paris, you might want to reconsider if you are at risk of forming a blood clot. If you are overweight, older than 50, or have had a prior history of a blood clot in either your leg or lungs, your risk of a blood clot forming in your leg and moving to your heart is increased. This blood clot traveling to your heart is known as a pulmonary embolism and can be fatal. Immobilization for long periods of time in the sitting position can increase your risk. Instead, drink extra water to stay hydrated and take hourly strolls up and down the aisle. While sitting, flex and extend your feet as if you were stepping on a gas pedal repeatedly ten times every hour.

72. Reserve a Bulkhead Seat

Even if you don't play basketball, the extra leg room in a first row bulkhead seat will give you more space to stretch out on your overnight flight. Before boarding, consider purchasing an inflatable pillow in the gift shop. You will find these pillows more comfortable than the ones available on your airplane. Enhanced comfort will likely increase the chance of getting restful sleep as you fly to your destination.

73. Get a Quiet Hotel Room

When traveling, call your hotel in advance to avert sleepless nights. Hotels com-monly have sleeping rooms next to elevators, above workout rooms, near ice machines. Make sure yours isn't one of them by calling ahead and asking for a room mid-hallway with rooms on both sides. You still run the risk of having to listen to someone's crying baby next door, but at least you've taken away the predictable disturbances.

74. Make Sure Your Hotel Room Is the Right Temperature

Check your temperature controls as soon as you get to your hotel room. Whether the hotel is a classic oldie or a brand new building, temperature controls can be confusing, stuck, or simply inaccurate. Immediately on entering the room, adjust the controls to your desired temperature and pay attention to the response. In some cases, when air conditioning or heating kicks on, the noise can rival the sound of a Jumbo Jet taking off. There may be nothing you can do about the noise aside from changing hotels, but at least you know what to expect and you'll be certain whether or not the controls do their job.

75. Block Out Unnecessary Light

Close the drapes in your hotel room to be sure they block out light completely. In your own home, you know whether or not you can see streetlights or a full moon from your bedroom window. Not so when you're on the road. To be sure that you don't have neon signs or lightning storms shocking you awake, be sure the drapes in your hotel room close properly and provide a solid block against any light.

76. Make Yourself at Home in the Hotel

Loss of sleep while you're on the road can be due to the strange environment. You are comfortable in your own surroundings, in your own bed. If you travel to the same city often, stay in the same hotel, and even the same room if that's possible. Otherwise, take steps to make the strange hotel space more familiar so that your brain can relax in the new environment. Listed below are a few ways to "trick" your senses into associating the foreign surroundings with home, or at least a relaxed state.

77. Know the Signs of Bedbugs

If you see something that looks like pepper or tiny rust-colored spots on the head-board of your bed or in the drapes, for example, ask for a room change. After ingesting blood, bed bugs excrete such dark dots, and even though the hotel may have brought in an exterminator so that what you see is an old problem, don't take chances. You don't have to move to another hotel, though, because it is not uncommon for a problem like this to be isolated.

78. Bring Your Favorite Smells with You

Bring your own shower gel if you have a favorite one. Sure, you get theirs for "free," but if it smells like lilies and you use a pomegranate/mango blend at home, then you may not find the lilies a peaceful scent.

79. Adhere to Your Bedtime Rituals on the Road

Regardless of whether it's doing a crossword puzzle, stretching, or calling your mom to say, "I love you," maintain your pre-sleep rituals when you travel. You have faith in them; your conditioned response is that you will sleep after you do them. In this way you can reduce anxiety about getting to sleep.

80. Bring Your Favorite Nighttime Drinks with You

If you normally drink chamomile tea or hot milk before bed at home, stick with your habit on the road if you can. Go to the dimly lit, quiet hotel bar and say, "Bartender, I'd like a glass of warm milk. Straight up." So many hotel rooms now have in-room coffee and tea service, you probably won't need to go to the bar or call room service. Pack your chamomile tea bags with your pajamas. Many hotels are now also getting savvy about this preference and routinely provide a few bags of "sleepy time tea" with their in-room coffee/tea service.

81. Make Sure That's Decaf

Without being rude, be sure your waiter gives you what you want. When you are out dining and the waiter begins to pour the coffee, be absolutely sure that what he is pouring is the caffeine free coffee that you requested. While it may seem impolite to ask a second time, you will be sorry you didn't when you return to your hotel and cannot fall asleep. If a restful night of sleep is important for that early morning meeting, you may want to skip even the "caffeine-free" coffee altogether.

82. Bring Snooze Music

Take snooze-inducing recordings with you. An increasing number of hotels are providing radio/CD players, and sometimes, the property will even have a selection of sleepy-time CDs in the gift shop if you forget yours. If you have a house by the ocean and can't sleep without the sound of waves breaking, then bring the sound with you.

83. Make Sure You Feel Safe

Double lock your door. While the chance of waking up to an intruder is remote, the fear of one might disrupt your sleep. Decrease this fear with the added security measure.

84. Find the Fire Exit

Know where the fire exit is on your floor. Most likely, you will never endure the trauma of a hotel fire. But knowing what the closest escape route is will give you peace of mind and more restful slumber.

85. Bring Your Own Alarm Clock

You have confidence in the functioning of your own clock. You don't want to wake up every hour with worries that the alarm clock in your hotel room is not going to wake you in time for your 6:00 A.M. flight. Pack your own clock and you'll have that added comfort.

86. Ask for a Wake-up Call

If you must be up at a certain time, call guest services to give you a wake-up call. While this backup to your alarm clock is likely unnecessary, it might give you the peace of mind you need so that you can sleep and not worry.

87. Continue Regular Exercise While on the Road

Someone who is used to physical exertion as part of a routine needs to continue that while traveling. Call your hotel or vacation spot ahead of time. Find out about workout facilities, pools, tennis courts, and jogging paths. If your hotel doesn't have the facilities you are accustomed to, ask about a local gym. You can also use exercise bands—easily packable—or a standard military workout of pushups, squats, dips, and running in place to keep yourself active so you sleep better.

88. Stay Hydrated at High Elevations

Drink extra water if you travel to a high elevation. A dramatic change in elevation can trigger altitude sickness, and one of the main symptoms is a headache that could easily keep you up at night. Rather than assume an aspirin alone will take care of it—it probably won't—keep yourself hydrated throughout the day and keep a glass of water next to you at night.

89. Climb the Mountain Slowly

At elevations above 8,000 feet, the chance of altitude sickness and sleep disruption increases. Allow your body time to acclimate by reaching higher elevations at a gradual pace.

90. Sleep at the Base of the Mountain

After your daily ascent to the mountaintop, sleeping at a lower elevation may lead to less sleep disruption related to high altitude. People who suddenly try to sleep at a high elevation often experience headaches and irregular breathing patterns that disrupt sleep.

91. Avoid Alcohol at High Elevations

Celebrate your journey with a non-alcoholic beverage. Alcohol consumption may magnify sleep disruption at higher elevations. It's more than just a matter of getting dried out—you may feel the effects of the alcohol a lot more and your hangover may be more memorable than your trip to the mountains.

92. Avoid Sunburns

Respect the sun at high elevations and use protection. Many people who come to the mountains think that the chill in the air somehow means that they won't get a burn from the sun. Quite the contrary. The effects of ultraviolet radiation at elevations around 8,000 feet and above can be shocking. People try to sleep and realize they feel as though they have spent the day on the beach in Mexico—unprotected.

93. Ask Your Physician about Acetazolamide

Symptoms of altitude sickness, including sleep disruption, may be decreased by the prophylactic use of acetazolamide. Don't take this medication if you are allergic to sulfa. The steroid, dexamethasone, is an alternative.

94. Call a Doctor If You Develop Extreme Sleepiness

Extreme sleepiness, lethargy, or difficulty breathing at a high altitude are all symptoms that may suggest potentially life threatening problems associated with high altitude. Pulmonary edema (buildup of fluid in the lungs) and cerebral edema (buildup of fluid in the brain) can occur. These are life-threatening problems that require immediate attention.

95. Check for Sleeping Sickness

Upon return from your safari in Africa, contact your physician with any new symptoms. Many different types of infections can be acquired on your trip—and they will disrupt your sleep. One potentially fatal illness is known as sleeping sickness. A bite from a tsetse fly can result in swollen glands, fever, and disrupted sleep, as well as excessive daytime sleepiness. Medical therapy is available. If any of these symptoms develop, seek immediate medical attention.

96. Check for Bacterial Infection and Parasites

If you experience gastrointestinal irritation after a trip—and it will disrupt your sleep—then get checked for a bacterial infection and parasites. The effect of having a bacterial infection or parasites, which are generally picked up from untreated water from both indoor and outdoor sources, can be that you just want to sleep to avoid the cramping and diarrhea. In this situation. do not seek relief with over-the-counter sleep medicines or alcohol, which do not address the underlying problem. See a physician: you may require medical treatment.

DRIVING

97. Get Enough Sleep Before You Drive

Sleeping well involves sleeping at the right location—and that rarely includes a car. Drowsiness is a major contributing factor to about 100,000 crashes a year, according to the National Highway Traffic Safety Administration of the US Department of Transportation, which also offers these eye-opening statistics:

- 1,500 deaths per year are a result of falling asleep at the wheel.
- 60 percent of Americans have driven while feeling sleepy.

- 37 percent of Americans have fallen asleep at the wheel within the past year.

To help counter the problem of driving while drowsy, the National Sleep Foundation (drowsydriving.org) has provided these tips, most of which will look familiar by now.

- Adult drivers should sleep seven to nine hours each night.
- Teenage drivers should sleep 8½ to 9½ hours each night.
- On long drives, take a break every two hours or every 100 miles.
- Drive with a friend or family member who can engage you in conversation and share the driving.
- Avoid alcohol.
- Avoid sedating drugs. Examples include antihistamines, benzodiazepines, and narcotics. Many other prescription drugs may also have sedation as a side effect.

98. Know the Signs of Drowsy Driving

Watch for the warning signs of drowsy driving, outlined by the National Sleep Foundation:

- Droopy, heavy eyelids
- Head nodding
- Yawning constantly
- Blurred vision

- Frequent blinking
- Daydreaming
- Trouble remembering last few miles
- Missing exits
- Unintentional veering out of your lane

99. Get a Room

Your body can tell it's time to get a good night's sleep. Heed the warning while driving, and pull over at a nearby motel or hotel. If this is not possible, drink coffee or other products containing caffeine and take a 15- to 20-minute nap in a safe place. It will take approximately 30 minutes for the caffeine to be absorbed into your system. During this period, napping will increase the likelihood that you will be able to drive more safely.

100. Late at Night, You Should Be Sleeping, Not Driving

The decreased visibility related to darkness, in combination with the inevitable drowsiness that occurs late at night, can be a fatal combination. If you must drive late, watch for warning signs as outlined above and take appropriate measures if you develop early signs of drowsiness.

101. Make Sure Your Teen Gets Enough Sleep Before Handing Over the Keys

Sleep deprivation, inexperience, and alcohol may be contributing factors to the fact that teenage drivers have big challenges when it comes to staying safe behind the wheel. Many teens do not get the 8½ to 9½ hours of sleep per night that are recommended for that age group. An accumulated sleep debt can be deadly for the young driver in your family.

102. Tell Your Parents You're Concerned about Their Driving If They Have Sleep Problems

Drive with your elderly parents or grandparents to see if they are driving safely. Changes in sleep architecture, medical conditions, and medications can contribute to daytime sleepiness in the elderly. Combine this with visual and hearing impairments that may occur as we get older, and you have a recipe for disaster. Share your concerns with your loved ones. When necessary, insist on doing the driving. Loss of independence with aging is difficult for many. Loss of driving privileges can be devastating. Remember, however, driving is a privilege and must be taken seriously by everyone in the family.

103. If You Drive a Bus or Truck, Society Depends on You to Be Alert

Watch for the warning signs of drowsiness and always practice good sleep hygiene measures. If you believe that you are suffering from one of the sleep disorders associated with daytime sleepiness discussed in this book, seek help immediately and stop driving. Talk to your physician or health care provider about seeing a sleep physician. While sleep centers often have waiting lists that can last many weeks, a direct call from your physician or health care provider to a sleep specialist detailing your history and your occupation will usually lead to an expedited evaluation. It is very likely that once you have been successfully treated, you will be able to return to your chosen occupation. However, make sure you wait until your sleep physician tells you it is safe to resume driving.

104. If You Work Twenty-Four Hours Straight, Sleep When You Get Home and Not While You're Driving

If you know you have to work twenty-four hours without a scheduled sleep period, plan ahead. Arrange for a friend or family member to drive you home or take public transportation. Your body will crave a good night's sleep at that point and the urge may be so overwhelming that you will not be able to overcome it.

ALLERGIES

105. Close Your Window During Allergy Season

Pollen can wreak havoc for many people. Even if you have no history of seasonal allergies, if you experience the onset of nasal congestion, a common symptom, then the pollen might be especially bad or you might not realize what new things have been planted outside your window. Nasal congestion will lead to decreased nasal airflow, snoring, and sleep disruption. It can worsen obstructive sleep apnea. If you experience difficulty breathing on spring and/or summer nights, just close the windows and turn on the air conditioner. What happens during the day should alert you to potential sleeping problems: Be mindful of this when symptoms such as stuffy nose and itchy and watery eyes occur.

106. Don't Overuse Over-the-Counter Nasal Sprays

Avoid repeated use of over-the-counter nasal sprays in your attempts to clear up congestion. While nasal steroids prescribed by a doctor can be extremely beneficial for allergy sufferers, over-the-counter nasal decongestants are a bad idea for more than three days in a row. They tend to cause a rebound effect so your problem gets worse instead of better.

107. Get a Prescription Nasal Spray

Ask your doctor for a prescription nasal spray you can use all during the allergy season. Nasal steroids can contribute to dramatic improvement of allergy symptoms because they decrease nasal inflammation and open the breathing passages. They also appear to be safe for long-term use. Additionally, nasal steroids may decrease the need for daytime antihistamines which can have a sedating effect.

108. Block Out Dust Mites

Invest in pillow casings that block dust mites to minimize allergic reactions. If you find yourself sniffling or coughing only at night, you might be battling mites. They are really common and invisible, so don't fire the housekeeper. Other allergens can also find good homes in your bedding and will cause a similar reaction if you have sensitivities. You can replace your pillows regularly, or take the more cost-effective route of getting a cover designed to provide a barrier between you and the allergen. These casings are also made for mattresses.

109. Lose the Feather Pillow

Do not use feather pillows if your eyes puff up at night or you have any other signs of allergy. Synthetic stuffing for pillows has improved so much that you no longer have to face the prospect of a lump of foam if you have allergies to feathers. Many people don't even know they're allergic to feathers until they wake up to puffy eyes in a nice hotel and blame the air, the carpet, or the wine they had the night before. Check your hotel room closet for "extra" pillows; they are probably stuffed with synthetic material. The fancy, down-stuffed ones are on the bed, ready to impress you and then make you sick. Call housekeeping and ask for replacements if you can't find them in the closet.

110. Invest in an Air Filter

Invest in an air filter if allergens continue to bother you. Allergens in the home such as dust and animal dander can be filtered through a HEPA filter, or a High Efficiency Particulate Air filter. You can buy them at stores or online. Place them in bedrooms to decrease allergy symptoms that include nasal stuffiness, coughing, and wheezing. This can help you breathe better and sleep better. If symptoms persist, see your doctor. You may need medical treatment for your allergies or asthma.

3

Advice for People Who
Sleep **Too Much**

111. Find Out If You're Sleep Deprived

112. Have Your Sleepiness Evaluated

113. Don't Blame Your Sleepiness on Age

114. Work with Your Teenaged Night Owl

115. Don't Worry If It's Harder to Stay Up Late as You Age

116. If Your Teen Has Episodic Sleepiness, Ask Your Doctor about a Very Rare Condition Known as Kleine-Levin Syndrome

117. With Intermittent Sleepiness, Look for Other Symptoms

118. If They Won't Wake Up, Call a Doctor

119. Get Extra Sleep During Your Period If It Wears You Out

120. Get Checked for Sleep Apnea

121. You May Have Narcolepsy If You Develop Sudden Uncontrollable Urges to Sleep

122. Seek Medical Evaluation for Sudden Episodes of Weakness

123. If You Have Daytime Sleepiness and Episodes of Paralysis at Night, You Should Be Evaluated for Narcolepsy

124. Consider the Possibility of Narcolepsy If You Have Hallucinations and Sleepiness

125. Pay Attention to Your Sleep–Wake Cycle If You Have Been Diagnosed with Narcolepsy

126. Seek Pharmaceutical Treatment If You Have Narcolepsy

127. Have Your Sleepy, Unfocused Teen Checked for Narcolepsy

128. If You Suspect That You Have Narcolepsy, You Need a Sleep Study

129. Ask about Idiopathic Hypersomnia

130. If You Are Still Sleepy After Being Treated for Sleep Apnea, You May Also Have Narcolepsy or Idiopathic Hypersomnia

131. If You Have a Sleep Disorder, Ask Your Physician for a Letter Documenting Your Condition

Sleeping "too much" on an occasional basis is common. Maybe the constant stress of a project at work is over and that leads to a long, luxurious sleep. Maybe you're on the verge of getting sick and your body just says, "I need a little more sleep today." Those are normal body responses, but these tips are about taking the right action if sleeping "too much" happens quite a bit.

111. Find Out If You're Sleep Deprived

If you think you are too sleepy during the daytime, you may not be getting enough sleep at night. There are a number of medical conditions that can cause you to be sleepy, but often the most obvious cause is overlooked. Modern society has found ways to lengthen the day and shorten the night, and the result is that many of us are sleep-deprived. If you sleep five to six hours per night during the week, and then find yourself sleeping much longer on the weekends, you may be in this category. The typical nightly sleep requirement is seven to nine hours, but there are some individuals who function well with less sleep ("short sleepers") and some who require more ("long sleepers"). These people are exceptional. Most of us who believe we are capable of normal daytime performance in spite of inadequate sleep would achieve much greater efficiency and productivity if we obtained more sleep.

112. Have Your Sleepiness Evaluated

Excessive sleepiness can have a variety of causes. In addition to the sleep disorders discussed in this book, medical conditions can be responsible for this symptom. In some cases, multiple sclerosis, stroke, head trauma, tumors, metabolic disorders, and other illnesses can cause increased sleepiness.

113. Don't Blame Your Sleepiness on Age

Brief daytime sleep episodes in the elderly are more common in sedentary situations if they have a sedentary lifestyle, but falling asleep at inappropriate times is not part of the normal aging process. Sometimes we assume that as people get older, sleepiness during inappropriate times is inevitable. This is not true and underlying conditions such as obstructive sleep apnea might be at fault. Seek medical evaluation if you notice a change in your level of alertness.

114. Work with Your Teenaged Night Owl

Sleepiness in adolescents may be due to a delayed sleep phase. Visit any college campus and you will see lights in the dormitories on half the night. Don't necessarily blame it on a teenager's first taste of freedom-from-parents or too much homework. This age group commonly has delayed sleep phase syndrome, in which the circadian rhythm shifts later by a few hours. Starting in the adolescent years, the body clock often undergoes a shift and "night owl" tendencies develop. Despite a 6:00 or 7:00 A.M. wake-up call, adolescents often seem unable to fall asleep until midnight or later. They become chronically sleep-deprived. They get to school late, feel sleepy during classes, and then come home and fight with everybody in sight. Some school districts in the United States have adopted later starting times for high schools in order to address this problem. If your teenaged offspring has a severely delayed sleep phase and is developing academic or social difficulty as a result, you should seek help from a sleep specialist.

115. Don't Worry If It's Harder to Stay Up Late as You Age

It is common for people to want to go to bed earlier as they get older. This change in sleep pattern advances the sleep phase. Individuals who retire to bed early and awaken early have advanced sleep phase syndrome. In this condition, the circadian rhythm moves in the opposite direction of the delayed sleep phase syndrome described above.

116. If Your Teen Has Episodic Sleepiness, Ask Your Doctor about a Very Rare Condition Known as Kleine-Levin Syndrome

This is a rare disorder, but it can cause episodes of sleepiness. The most common occurrence is in adolescent boys, who may have several bouts of sleepiness and irritability lasting days to weeks occurring at variable intervals over the course of several years. During these periods there may be an increase in appetite and sexual behavior. The cause of this disorder is unknown, and treatment is often ineffective. Fortunately, the episodes seem to disappear after several years. Females as well as males can be affected.

117. With Intermittent Sleepiness, Look for Other Symptoms

Other causes of episodic sleepiness include a form of migraine headache known as basilar migraine, and mood disturbances. Symptoms of basilar migraine can include vertigo and visual problems. Symptoms of a mood disturbance can include feelings of sadness, guilt, worthlessness, changes in eating patterns and the inability to make decisions. Depression can lead to chronic fatigue, but bipolar illness, with its cycling highs and lows, can cause episodic sleepiness alternating with periods of insomnia. In all cases, these are conditions that need medical attention, not home remedies.

118. If They Won't Wake Up, Call a Doctor

Seek immediate medical attention if a relative or friend is suddenly so sleepy that they cannot be aroused to their normal level of consciousness. Remember that sleep is a fully reversible state. Severe life threatening infections in the lung or urinary tract, or electrolyte abnormalities are common causes of sudden changes in mental status, particularly in the elderly. These are emergencies requiring immediate medical attention.

119. Get Extra Sleep During Your Period If It Wears You Out

Take some extra time to sleep if your menstrual period wears you out. During their reproductive years, women can experience significant sleepiness during their period. If possible, adjust your schedule to allow time for naps and maybe an early-to-bed regimen.

120. Get Checked for Sleep Apnea

Endless drowsy days could signal the presence of sleep apnea. If you know you snore loudly or have gained weight, your sleepiness may be due to sleep apnea. Sleep apnea affects as many as 4 percent of middle-aged women and 9 percent of middle-aged men. It is discussed in detail in Chapter 6: Advice for People Who Snore.

121. You May Have Narcolepsy If You Develop Sudden Uncontrollable Urges to Sleep

Narcolepsy is a neurologic disorder, and the most prominent symptom is excessive sleepiness. People who have narcolepsy fall asleep in a variety of inappropriate situations. Sometimes, they have a sense of being drowsy; at other times, sleep takes over suddenly. Narcoleptics typically find brief naps refreshing. Narcolepsy can cause a number of other symptoms as well. These additional symptoms are covered in the next few paragraphs.

122. Seek Medical Evaluation for Sudden Episodes of Weakness

Weakness can have many causes. A specific type of weakness called cataplexy can be seen in patients with narcolepsy. Cataplexy is defined as brief episodes of muscular weakness, and is usually triggered by laughter or other strong emotions. Severe episodes of cataplexy may lead to a fall, but there can be subtler forms of weakness such as knee buckling, or drooping of the head or jaw. Cataplexy generally lasts for seconds, and patients remain awake during the episodes. Not all patients who are given a diagnosis of narcolepsy have cataplexy.

123. If You Have Daytime Sleepiness and Episodes of Paralysis at Night, You Should Be Evaluated for Narcolepsy

Episodes of paralysis lasting seconds that occur when falling asleep or waking up are called sleep paralysis. Sleep paralysis can be frightening to patients, but the episodes resolve spontaneously and do not pose a threat to breathing.

124. Consider the Possibility of Narcolepsy If You Have Hallucinations and Sleepiness

Hallucinations as you fall asleep or wake up might also be due to narcolepsy. These hallucinations represent the intrusion of REM sleep dream imagery into wakefulness. Like cataplexy and sleep paralysis, conditions in which the muscle paralysis of REM sleep appears at the wrong time, these hallucinations illustrate the fact that in narcolepsy the normal control of the sleep-wake cycle is impaired.

125. Pay Attention to Your Sleep–Wake Cycle If You Have Been Diagnosed with Narcolepsy

Sleeping poorly at night, combined with overwhelming sleepiness during the daytime, could also signal narcolepsy, so get an evaluation. Disruption of the sleep-wake cycle in narcolepsy can produce fragmented sleep at night. It may seem puzzling that patients who are excessively sleepy also complain of poor sleep at night, but narcolepsy affects people around the clock. Sleepiness intrudes into wakefulness and wakefulness intrudes into sleep.

126. Seek Pharmaceutical Treatment If You Have Narcolepsy

The sleepiness of narcolepsy can be treated with conventional stimulants like methylphenidate and dextroamphetamine. However, modafinil and armodafinil promote wakefulness with fewer side effects and less abuse potential than the older medications. Cataplexy can be treated with alerting antidepressants such as fluoxetine and venlafaxine which suppress REM sleep. Sodium oxybate, a liquid medication taken at night, can be used to treat both sleepiness and cataplexy.

127. Have Your Sleepy, Unfocused Teen Checked for Narcolepsy

Symptoms of narcolepsy typically develop in the teens or twenties. This is a time of life when many individuals obtain insufficient sleep. It is also not uncommon for attention deficit disorder (ADD) or ADHD (attention deficit hyperactivity disorder) to be diagnosed in adolescence. Teenagers who have trouble concentrating or staying awake may need to be evaluated for narcolepsy before the label of ADD is applied, and before it is assumed that sleepiness is simply due to sleep deprivation.

128. If You Suspect That You Have Narcolepsy, You Need a Sleep Study

If narcolepsy is suspected as a diagnosis, you should undergo a sleep study. The diagnosis of narcolepsy is made with an overnight sleep study followed by a daytime sleep study called a Multiple Sleep Latency Test. The overnight study enables sleep physicians to rule out sleep apnea and other nocturnal disturbances that might cause daytime sleepiness. The Multiple Sleep Latency Test consists of a series of five twenty-minute nap opportunities that allow physicians to measure how quickly patients fall asleep and to determine whether or not they enter REM sleep when they do so. Patients who fall asleep on average in 8 minutes or less, and who enter REM sleep in at least two naps, have findings consistent with narcolepsy.

129. Ask about Idiopathic Hypersomnia

If your tests do not show narcolepsy or sleep apnea, you may be someone with idiopathic hypersomnia. You would have no symptoms of cataplexy or exhibit any tendency to enter REM sleep during the daytime. Unlike narcoleptics, you would not report vivid dreams. You would not usually find sleep refreshing, and may have a great deal of difficulty in arising in the morning. Like narcolepsy, idiopathic hypersomnia is generally treated with conventional stimulants or modafinil.

130. If You Are Still Sleepy After Being Treated for Sleep Apnea, You May Also Have Narcolepsy or Idiopathic Hypersomnia

Sleep apnea (discussed in the chapter giving tips to people who snore) is one of the most commonly diagnosed sleep disorders. Patients who remain sleepy despite successful treatment for sleep apnea may have another cause. If you fall into this category, ask your physician to re-evaluate you for an additional cause of your symptoms. You may need treatment with stimulant medication or modafinil. This is sometimes necessary even if no additional diagnosis can be made in order to relieve residual sleepiness in patients with treated sleep apnea.

131. If You Have a Sleep Disorder, Ask Your Physician for a Letter Documenting Your Condition

You may feel a great sense of relief once your physician tells you that your sleepiness is due to a treatable medical condition. However, your employer may have already criticized your work ethic, "written you up," passed you over for promotion, or given you a stern warning. Ask your physician or health care provider to construct a thoughtful letter explaining your medical condition and its impact on your work. Reasonable accommodations at work should be discussed. Give your physician permission to talk directly with your boss if necessary. Don't hesitate to talk to someone in human resources or to your union representative if your boss is not sympathetic.

4

Advice for People Who Sleep
at the **Wrong Time**

132. Allow Yourself Adequate Time to Sleep

133. Try to Keep the Same Schedule

134. When You're Faced with the Prospect of Rotating Shifts, Consider What Impact It Will Have on Your Sleep

135. Adjust Your Light Exposure

136. Adjust Your Sound Exposure

137. Watch for Weight Gain

138. Use Light Therapy

139. You Can Benefit from Evening Light if You Want to Delay Bedtime

140. Research Melatonin

141. Ask for Help If You're a New Mother

142. Sleep When the Baby Sleeps

143. Have Emergency Response Ready for Elderly Relatives

144. Share Care-Giving Responsibilities

"Wrong time" refers both to sleeping out of synch with the typical circadian rhythm out of necessity—usually a job or care-giving responsibilities, or due to innate shifts in your own circadian rhythm.

From a medical perspective, one of the topics that would normally be addressed in this chapter is jet lag, but in this book, we have included it with the other tips on traveling that appear in Chapter 2.

In this chapter, we offer tips for shift workers and caregivers, as well as for people with unusual body clocks. If you're a caregiver to a baby or young children, you will also want to see Chapter 5: Advice for People with Kids.

SHIFT WORKERS

132. Allow Yourself Adequate Time to Sleep

Shift workers need to recognize the sleep drive, not ignore it. For shift workers, sleep in the daytime is often not very effective. There is an inclination to minimize the need for sleep because daytime provides the best opportunity to shop, keep doctors' appointments, garden, and complete other household chores. Your first step to getting restful sleep is to acknowledge that you must alter your circadian rhythm, and that means you must minimize your obligations during the day; it's your sacred bedtime.

133. Try to Keep the Same Schedule

Try to keep the same schedule if you are a shift worker. Changing shifts frequently confuses your brain as to whether it's time to be awake or asleep. If you have the option of sticking to a single shift, do it, or at the very least, stick to a single shift for as long as you can. Also, try to maintain the schedule of sleeping during the day and being up at night when you're off. You're thinking: "That's impossible!" and you're probably right unless you have no family and want to do all of your shopping over the internet at midnight. All we're saying is that maintaining the schedule is ideal for sleep.

134. When You're Faced with the Prospect of Rotating Shifts, Consider What Impact It Will Have on Your Sleep

If your shifts change, try to go from day to evening to night. It's easier for people to stay up later and later than it is to do the reverse.

135. Adjust Your Light Exposure

Adjust your light exposure to support your being awake at night and asleep during the day. Light is one example of what sleep specialists call a "zeitgeiber," literally, a time giver. Control light exposure and you can fool your brain into thinking that night is day and day is night. Here are three primary ways to do that: 1. Invest in opaque drapes, a blindfold, or whatever is necessary to block the light while you're trying to sleep. 2. Wear sunglasses home from work after your night shift so that you minimize exposure to full daylight. 3. Give yourself continual exposure to the lights of your workplace, rather than sneaking off to a dark broom closet when you take a break.

136. Adjust Your Sound Exposure

Adjust your sound exposure to support your being awake at night and asleep during the day. Sound is another zeitgeiber. If you associate the noise of traffic with daytime and silence with night, then your brain will not want to sleep when you hear honking horns and screeching tires. You need the cooperation of people around you to shut down the noise. In addition to doing what you personally can to block disruptive sounds, ask your family to turn off the ringer on the phones, and let your neighbors know that you work the night shift so they are less likely to mow the grass close to your bedroom window on a weekday. If you can afford noise-canceling headsets, invest in them. Here's an idea: Get those family members and neighbors who want to make noise during the day to pool their money and buy you one of those top-of-the-line noise canceling headsets for your birthday.

137. Watch for Weight Gain

Watch for weight gain if you're a shift worker. Sleep deprivation may be a risk factor for obesity. Leptin is a hormone that lowers appetite. There is evidence that sleep deprivation lowers your leptin levels. Your appetite may remain high and you may gain weight as a result. And if you're sleepy, you tend to eat more to stay awake, so you are trapped in a vicious cycle. If you've recently started shift work and notice a weight gain, it may be more than those trips to the vending machine adding some inches and pounds. Your body might also be telling you it needs more quality sleep.

138. Use Light Therapy

Use light therapy if you have a job that starts at 9:00 A.M., but you wake up at noon. Theater people who love their wake/work hours of 10:00 A.M. to 2:00 A.M., as well as shift workers who are happiest with a 4:00 P.M.–midnight schedule, are examples of those whose natural rhythm reflects a delayed sleep phase. Like teenagers with a delayed sleep phase, such people are night owls. This may not be a problem for those who work in the evenings and go to bed after midnight, but night owls have difficulty in coping with a more typical work or school schedule. That 8:00 A.M. physics class will never start at 11:00 just to accommodate a class full of bleary-eyed 19-year-olds. And that office job that starts a month after four years of cutting early classes to sleep in won't last long if your brain doesn't get into gear until noon. Every day, it's the same thing: tired, depressed, cranky, headachey. What allows you to change your biorhythm? Light. There is a pathway from the retina to the part of the brain that is responsible for your circadian rhythm. With the help of a sleep specialist, you can try to shift your circadian rhythm by using a light box that emits 5,000–10,000 lux (the unit describing the level of luminescence). The device, which emits light similar to sunlight, but without the ultraviolet radiation, will help you reset your internal clock. There is some evidence that blue light may be particularly effective. Early morning light exposure for at least thirty minutes is required to help advance the sleep phase. The best time to obtain morning light exposure depends on your sleep schedule, and this is where the advice of a sleep physician may be particularly helpful. The benefit is that it will send a message to the brain that says, "Hey! It's time to get up—now!" Light exposure at the right time can gradually shift the circadian rhythm to what many people consider normal (or at least what your boss considers normal). But if you don't have to begin the day at 7:00 A.M., then enjoy your biorhythm as it is.

139. You Can Benefit from Evening Light If You Want to Delay Bedtime

If you are a "lark" rather than a night owl, you could improve your social life with a light box. If your tendency is to retire to bed in the early evening hours and awaken before dawn, your circadian rhythm is advanced. It is shifted in the opposite direction from that of the person with a sleep phase delay. The advanced sleep phase usually does not interfere with employment; in fact it may be advantageous if you are a farmer. But it may limit social activity in the evening. Treatment, when necessary, can be accomplished with a light box, but patients with advanced sleep phase need light exposure in the evening rather than in the morning.

140. Research Melatonin

If you are being treated for a delayed sleep phase, ask your physician about the role of melatonin. Morning light exposure is necessary to combat a delayed sleep phase. Melatonin can also be a helpful tool in shifting the circadian rhythm. Just as light helps to inform the body clock that it is time to wake up, melatonin may notify the body clock that it is bedtime. The combined effects of melatonin at night and light exposure in the morning can be the most effective way to address your night owl tendencies. Be sure to discuss the timing and dosage of melatonin with your sleep physician, and discuss the timing of light exposure as well.

CAREGIVERS

141. Ask for Help If You're a New Mother

It not only takes a village to raise a child, but also to get good sleep after you've had the baby. Sleep architecture changes for new parents. You will hear them say things like, "I can sleep through a tornado, but if my baby is kicking in the crib, I'll hear it." Just after delivery, mothers spend less time in deep sleep, which makes sense from an evolutionary perspective. Mothers particularly are likely to be more easily awakened than before the birth so they can be prepared to battle the wolves at the door. Not getting a good night's sleep can magnify the feelings of depression and anger that follow childbirth for many women. New mothers should identify friends and family members who are candidates for babysitting for at least two hours so you can get a nap, go to the gym, or sit in the bathtub.

142. Sleep When the Baby Sleeps

If you're home alone with a new baby, sleep when the baby sleeps. The baby will sleep about half the time, so you can get plenty of opportunities to indulge as well. Since it's unrealistic to assume that you will get an uninterrupted eight hours of sleep a night, take it when you can get it.

143. Have Emergency Response Ready for Elderly Relatives

Put an emergency response system in place with your elderly relatives so you can get some sleep. Having elderly parents or other close relatives who wish to remain in their own home—no matter what—presents huge stresses. Nighttime, when the elderly are more likely to fall going to the bathroom, is a particularly dangerous time. You lose sleep over the worry and find yourself cat-napping at work to make up for it. You can take action by calling an emergency response system provider like Life Alert and make it more affordable by taking advantage of discounts offered through organizations like AARP.

144. Share Care-Giving Responsibilities

Organize yourself to be able to share caregiving. Peace of mind that the details of care-giving are in place goes a long way to helping you rest well. Put a little package together for your helpers, whether they are paid or unpaid, so they can share care-giving responsibilities for an elderly relative. It should contain insurance information, social security number, extra keys to the car and house, basic information about medical history and conditions, a list of current medications and when they must be taken, and the names and numbers of key physicians.

5

Advice for People with **Kids**

145. Develop a Sleep Routine for Your Child

146. Inform the Babysitter about the Sleep Routine

147. Stick to the Routine

148. Set Limits

149. Establish Familiarity in the Child's Bedroom

150. Keep Environmental Elements as Consistent as Possible

151. Consider the Downsides of Co-Sleeping

152. Don't Skip the Naps

153. Sleep Begets Sleep, so Try to Solve Your Child's Bedtime Problems with a Nap

154. Check Family History of Bedwetting

155. Don't Overreact to Sleepwalking

156. Create an Alert System When Your Sleepwalker Walks

157. If You Were a Sleepwalker, or Already Have One Child Who Sleepwalks, Keep an Eye on Your Other Kids

158. Observe a Child with Night Terrors, but Do Not Try to Wake Him

159. Get Your Snoring Child Checked for Enlarged Tonsils

160. If Your Child Can't Stop Eating, Have Your Health Care Provider Check for Prader-Willi Syndrome

Here is a series of tips that will help parents with newborns through the pre-adolescent stages. If your child experiences episodes of sleepwalking or night terrors, in addition to the tips in this section, you will also want to get a more thorough understanding of such parasomnias by going through Chapter 7.

145. Develop a Sleep Routine for Your Child

Predictability works well in teaching a child to sleep through the night. It's reassuring to the child and establishes if-then expectations, such as if pajamas go on, then bedtime comes soon afterward. Look at your own schedule as part of the set-up for your child's bedtime. You have dinner, clean up, and then start the preparation for bedtime. The sequence of events then moves to the moment when it's time to climb into bed.

146. Inform the Babysitter about the Sleep Routine

Tell anyone who puts the child to bed what the sleep routine is. Part of your child's sleep routine might be singing a song, reading a book, saying prayers, and other nighttime rituals, so be sure to tell the babysitter what all of the pieces in the sequence are. It's important that the babysitter not lose track of time, too, since it's not just the routine that matters, but when the routine occurs.

147. Stick to the Routine

Stick to the sleep routine no matter how "cruel" it seems. Establishing a bedtime sequence of events reinforces expectations of a positive nighttime experience for your child, and deviations from this sequence may give rise to behavioral insomnia of childhood, which involves the development of habits or associations that make it difficult for a child to fall asleep or get back to sleep. This is why it's important to know what the routine should and should not involve; you could be starting a habit or association that could be very hard to undo. One of the elements of a healthy routine is having the child in the bed when he's ready for sleep, as opposed to letting him fall asleep on the couch in front of the TV and then carrying him to bed. Another variation—and this is a hard one for parents to let go—is staying in the child's bedroom and lying next to him until he's asleep or reading until he's fallen asleep. You want to help the child calm down, but also help him learn to soothe himself to sleep. If your child has grown accustomed to your being there every night until he drifts off, then the evening you have something else to do, that child will likely have real problems sleeping well.

148. Set Limits

Set limits on what the sleep routine involves. Children can be artful procrastinators and manipulators. If you usually read one book before bedtime, how easy would it be to get you to read two? Or three? Suddenly the routine has expanded considerably. Just say no. Otherwise, you might find that after the third book, they want a sip of water, and then a cough drop, and then an extra blanket, and before you know it, your spouse is asleep and you haven't even finished loading the dishwasher. Establish limits with the big things like no TV after a certain hour, as well as the small ones like an extra book.

149. Establish Familiarity in the Child's Bedroom

Arrange the sleeping situation and stay with the scheme for a while. Introducing new mobiles and wall hangings and giant stuffed animals may be a good idea for a playroom, but it's better to keep the bedroom décor more stable than that.

150. Keep Environmental Elements as Consistent as Possible

We all wake up at various times of the night because of sleep cycles and children are no different. If your child goes to bed with a nightlight on in the hall, but the nightlight is off when he awakens briefly during the night, that difference could be enough to make it hard to get back to sleep. The same could be true for music playing softly that cuts off at a certain time. Give some consideration to ambient lights and sounds that your child is likely to associate with bedtime and respect how their sudden absence could create a temporary problem.

151. Consider the Downsides of Co-Sleeping

Consider the downsides of co-sleeping with your child before you make a habit of it. Although some cultures value having young children sleep in the same bed as the parents, make a personal decision about this based on safety, as well as psychology and sleep requirements. Infants have died as a result of a sleeping parent rolling over on the baby; this is particularly possible when parent and baby fall asleep together in an easy chair. Parents also risk a loss of their

own intimacy if a child or children sleep with them. The bed might ev
crowded that one of the parents will just sleep in the child's room to be able to
stretch out.

152. Don't Skip the Naps

Sleep is important for memory and learning, and as young children are developing—and they do so rapidly—the nap supports healthy development. Some kids who show signs of attention deficit hyperactivity disorder are actually sleep deprived. On a less severe scale, they might just be cranky and impatient as a result of inadequate sleep.

153. Sleep Begets Sleep, so Try to Solve Your Child's Bedtime Problems with a Nap

Some parents face a child's nighttime difficulty with a paradoxical solution: They push bedtime later, thinking that the child will get so sleepy that putting him down will be a cinch. What actually happens is that many children have greater difficulty sleeping when they are sleep deprived. The strategy backfires. Adding a nap may improve the child's ability to fall asleep at night.

154. Check Family History of Bedwetting

Check your own history if your child is a bed wetter, a problem that can interrupt sleep for both child and parents. Children are generally dry by the time they are seven, and many are dry before that. But before panicking and anticipating that you'll have to put waterproof protectors on your kid's bed until he's a teen, look at your own history. Was dad a bed wetter until he was eight or nine? This late-bloomer tendency can be hereditary. If, on the other hand, bedwetting remains a problem, seek advice from your pediatrician.

155. Don't Overreact to Sleepwalking

Gently guide your sleepwalking child back to bed. Overreacting to a sleepwalker's actions is not a good idea. Observe your child to be sure she's safe, but don't frighten her awake. Basic motor skills are still intact in this state, so she'll be able to walk down stairs, for example. (Also see Chapter 7: Advice for People with Odd Behaviors During Sleep.)

156. Create an Alert System When Your Sleepwalker Walks

Put a little bell on your sleepwalking child's door, or use some other non-intrusive alert. In most cases, you should have nothing to worry about with a sleepwalking child, but you may wish to be alerted if he or she leaves the bedroom. If your child has attempted to leave the house via a door or window, you should make sure that these exits are secured.

157. If You Were a Sleepwalker, or Already Have One Child Who Sleepwalks, Keep an Eye on Your Other Kids

This kind of behavior tends to run in families, so if you were a sleepwalker, or one of your children was a sleepwalker, siblings may have the same problem.

158. Observe a Child with Night Terrors, but Do Not Try to Wake Him

The challenge for parents who have a child experiencing night terrors is to do nothing except observe the child and make sure he doesn't harm himself. The next morning, that child will have no signs of psychological trauma from the episode, but he may if mom and dad screamed and tried to force him to wake up.

159. Get Your Snoring Child Checked for Enlarged Tonsils

The most common cause for sleep apnea in children is enlarged tonsils and the cure is tonsillectomy. Sometimes, a deformity or an inherited anatomical abnormality will also cause sleep apnea. A recessed jaw is one possible inherited cause. Children with Down Syndrome may suffer from obstructive sleep apnea because of the jaw anatomy generally associated with this condition.

160. If Your Child Can't Stop Eating, Have Your Health Care Provider Check for Prader-Willi Syndrome

Prader-Willi syndrome is a rare genetic disorder characterized by excessive food ingestion due to a decreased ability to sense being full. If food ingestion is not carefully monitored and limited, severe obesity and, consequently, obstructive sleep apnea can develop. Children with Prader-Willi syndrome often have an intellectual disability. Genetic tests can establish the diagnosis. Long-term treatment requires controlling access to food, usually under the watchful eye of a family member.

6

Advice for People Who **Snore**

161. Have Your Snoring Evaluated

162. Be Cautious Taking Narcotics If You Snore

163. You May Want to Avoid Sedatives If You Snore

164. Use Alcohol Moderately

165. Protect Your Nose If You're an Athlete

166. Find Out If You Have Primary Snoring

167. Find Out If You Have Upper Airway Resistance Syndrome

168. Find Out If You Have Obstructive Sleep Apnea

169. Remember That Sleep Apnea Becomes More Common as We Age

170. Know the Signs Of Sleep Apnea

171. Get Checked for Obesity Hypoventilation Syndrome

172. Measure the Size of Your Neck

173. No Matter What Your Weight, Check with Your Doctor about Your Airway Anatomy

174. If You Have a Small Jaw or Receding Chin and Snore Loudly, Find Out If You Have Sleep Apnea

175. If You're Pregnant, Don't Ignore Snoring

176. If You Have a Child with Down Syndrome, Ask Your Doctor about Sleep Apnea

177. If You Have Atrial Fibrillation, Ask If Sleep Apnea Is Causing It

178. Symptoms of Sleep Apnea Mean You Need a Sleep Study

179. Know What to Expect During a Sleep Study

180. You Do Not Need to Sleep Soundly During Your Sleep Study

181. If You Find It Hard to Relax in Unfamiliar Situations, Ask If You Can Take a Sleeping Pill to Get You Through Your Sleep Study

182. Try to Sleep on Your Back and Your Side During Your Sleep Study

183. After Your Sleep Study, Ask about Sleep Stages and Other Findings in Addition to Changes in Breathing

184. Determine Your "Sleep Efficiency"

185. Find Out Whether You Were Seen in All Sleep Stages

186. Ask If You Exhibited "Alpha-Delta" Sleep

187. Ask Whether Your Periodic Limb Movements Really Need to Be Treated

188. After Your Sleep Study, Work with Your Physician to Find an Appropriate Treatment for Your Snoring or Sleep Apnea

189. If You Have Insomnia or an Unusual Schedule, Keep a Sleep Log Before Your Visit with a Sleep Physician

206. Get the Right Surgeon to Perform Your Snore-Aid Procedures

207. Don't Hesitate to Try a Nasal CPAP Machine

208. Identify the CPAP Mask or Facial Attachment That You Find Most Comfortable

209. Add Humidity to the Process If You Have Nasal Stuffiness When Using CPAP

210. Lower the CPAP Pressure

211. Try Adaptive Servo-Ventilation

212. Be Honest about the Amount of Time You Use CPAP

213. Bring Your CPAP with You on Your Vacation

214. Try Bilevel Pressure

215. Try APAP

216. Prior to Surgery, Tell Your Doctor If You Have Sleep Apnea

217. If You Have Severe Obstructive Sleep Apnea, Find Out If You Need a Pacemaker

218. Take Your CPAP to the Hospital If You're Admitted

219. Get an Echocardiogram After Your Sleep Apnea Is Treated

220. Get Checked for Cushing's Syndrome

221. Get Checked for Acromegaly

222. Get Checked for Polycythemia

223. Ask Your Physician about Obstructive Sleep Apnea as a Cause of Protein in Your Urine

Snoring is common. It may be simply an annoyance, or it may be a symptom of obstructive sleep apnea, which is a potentially serious medical condition. In this chapter we discuss the spectrum of breathing abnormalities that can occur during sleep, as well as the treatments for everything from "just" snoring to the really serious health conditions that involve snoring.

161. Have Your Snoring Evaluated

Snoring may require a medical evaluation. There are potentially three levels of obstruction in the airway that can contribute to snoring problems. These areas include the nasal passage, the area behind the palate, and the area behind the tongue. An ear, nose and throat specialist can easily check you with a fiberoptic scope to help determine if an anatomic abnormality is contributing to airway obstruction. Causes could include enlarged tonsils, a swollen uvula or turbinates (ridges in the nose), an unusually large tongue, excessive tissue in the back of the throat, or a deviated nasal septum. Anatomic airway abnormalities as described above can contribute to a wide spectrum of disorders known as sleep-disordered breathing.

162. Be Cautious Taking Narcotics If You Snore

Narcotic pain relievers prescribed by physicians can worsen snoring and cause apneas due to relaxation of airway muscles in the back of your throat.

163. You May Want to Avoid Sedatives If You Snore

If you snore, be careful with sedatives such as benzodiazepines. Benzodiazepines prescribed for sleep or anxiety can worsen snoring or cause apneas due to relaxation of airway muscles in the back of the throat.

164. Use Alcohol Moderately

Even people who don't normally snore sometimes do when they drink, so be careful with alcohol. Alcohol ingestion can worsen snoring and cause apneas due to relaxation of airway muscles in the back of your throat.

165. Protect Your Nose If You're an Athlete

Athletes, protect your nose. Those of you competing in contact sports such as football, boxing, or hockey will be at risk for nasal trauma. Structural changes in your nasal anatomy can obstruct airflow. This may lead to snoring and obstructive sleep apnea. Surgery may become necessary to improve your nasal airflow.

166. Find Out If You Have Primary Snoring

If you snore without any interruption in your breathing during sleep, you have primary snoring, and you can take action to alleviate it. You may get complaints, but primary snoring usually will not disrupt your sleep or cause daytime symptoms.

167. Find Out If You Have Upper Airway Resistance Syndrome

Snoring that becomes progressively louder and causes you to awaken is reason to tell your doctor. This is more worrisome than primary snoring. With this condition, called Upper Airway Resistance Syndrome, crescendo snoring is associated with sleep disruption and excessive daytime sleepiness, but there is no significant collapse of the airway.

168. Find Out If You Have Obstructive Sleep Apnea

If you or others suspect that you actually stop breathing during sleep, you may have obstructive sleep apnea and definitely need to see your doctor. With this condition, in addition to snoring, the progressive relaxation of the airway muscles leads to partial collapse (hypopnea) or complete collapse (apnea) of the airway. Millions of Americans have obstructive sleep apnea, but only an estimated one tenth of them are aware of it. Everyone's upper airway muscles lose tone during sleep as muscles relax. The effect may be most pronounced in REM sleep. For people with sleep apnea, the airway muscles and the back of the tongue relax into a closed position and breathing stops. First, there is snoring, and then as the airway gets narrower and narrower, airflow is blocked. The brain senses the collapse, the loss of airflow and associated drop in blood oxygen level and sends a message to the airway to open up. Eventually, the airway responds and air rushes in. But this brain activity causes a brief arousal, and frequent apnea is therefore very disruptive to sleep. Sleep in people with apnea is typically not refreshing even if they are in bed for eight hours. Untreated sleep apnea increases the risk of hypertension, heart attack and irregular heart rhythms, elevated blood sugar, and stroke. Sleep apnea also poses huge dangers to society because someone who isn't well rested can fall asleep or "fade away" at inopportune times—while driving, operating a fork lift, giving airplanes clearance to land, or pushing buttons at a nuclear power plant. Excessive daytime sleepiness is a hallmark of someone affected by sleep apnea. CPAP, the most effective treatment for patients with sleep apnea, is discussed later in this section.

169. Remember That Sleep Apnea Becomes More Common as We Age

Although obstructive sleep apnea in non-elderly people is often linked to obesity, it is not necessarily associated with being overweight for elderly people. With aging, there are often changes in the anatomy of the airway that predispose a person to obstructive sleep apnea. As everything in the facial area, from eyelids to earlobes, begins to sag, the tone of the airway muscles can also decrease with aging. A doctor can help you with sleep apnea at any age, so don't just live with it. By the way, there is a hypothesis that Australian aborigines who play the didgeridoo may have less obstructive sleep apnea because of the toning effect of playing this long (up to almost 10 feet) wind instrument on the airways. Maybe it's time for a new hobby.

170. Know the Signs of Sleep Apnea

The American Academy of Sleep Medicine suggests a number of criteria to help determine whether or not a person may be suffering from obstructive sleep apnea. Check for these signs, and if you are not sure you have them, then ask your sleeping partner for input. Once you have a suspicion that you may have sleep apnea, your first step to getting a good night's sleep is to get medical help because the final piece of the diagnosis should be confirmed with a sleep study. Worrisome signs or symptoms include the following:

- Witnessed periods of not breathing
- Choking or gasping at night
- Recurrent awakenings from loud, disruptive snoring
- Sleep that you don't find refreshing
- Daytime fatigue
- Decreased concentration
- Excessive daytime sleepiness
- Morning headaches
- Decreased memory

If any of these symptoms occur, you might be at risk for heart attack or stroke. While the peak hours for sudden cardiac death in the general population are between 6:00 A.M. and noon, the peak hours for sudden cardiac death in sleep apnea patients is between midnight and 6:00 A.M. during the sleeping hours.

171. Get Checked for Obesity Hypoventilation Syndrome

If you are morbidly obese and experience daytime sleepiness, you may have obesity hypoventilation syndrome (OHS)—a compelling reason to seek medical help. This is the fourth, and most serious, level on the spectrum of sleep disordered breathing. These patients are at serious risk for death due to cardio-vascular collapse. Fatal cardiac arrhythmias may occur. Characteristic findings in these patients include morbid obesity, profound daytime sleepiness, swollen reddened legs, and congestive heart failure.

172. Measure the Size of Your Neck

Large necks are associated with an increased chance that you have obstructive sleep apnea. As you have deposited fat around your neck, you have likely also deposited fat inside your throat. Just a few extra millimeters of fat can narrow your airway significantly. Relaxation of airway muscles during sleep can lead to airway collapse and apnea. For women, a collar size greater than sixteen is asso-ciated with an increased incidence of obstructive sleep apnea. For men, a collar size greater than seventeen is associated with an increased incidence of obstruc-tive sleep apnea. While a large neck size alone does not signify the presence of obstructive sleep apnea, the presence of other symptoms as outlined would certainly raise a concern.

173. No Matter What Your Weight, Check with Your Doctor about Your Airway Anatomy

You do not have to be obese to have Obstructive Sleep Apnea. While the majority of patients with snoring, upper airway resistance syndrome, and obstructive sleep apnea are overweight, people with normal weight can certainly develop these problems as well. In the non-obese patient with sleep-disordered breathing, it may be due to obstructive problems in the nose and throat or changes in facial structure (see the next entry).

174. If You Have a Small Jaw or Receding Chin and Snore Loudly, Find Out If You Have Sleep Apnea

A small jaw lessens the size of the airway and makes it more likely that the airway will collapse when throat muscles relax.

175. If You're Pregnant, Don't Ignore Snoring

You should not pass off snoring during pregnancy as "one of those annoying things." There is an increased incidence of obstructive sleep apnea associated with pregnancy. It may be related to weight gain as well as fluid retention contributing to swelling in the airway. Untreated obstructive sleep apnea may have a negative impact on the health of the mother in terms of high blood pressure, and on the developing infant in terms of oxygen delivery and development.

176. If You Have a Child with Down Syndrome, Ask Your Doctor about Sleep Apnea

If you have a child with Down Syndrome and notice sleeping problems, ask your pediatrician about sleep apnea. Particular facial structures can increase the risk of sleep apnea. People with Down Syndrome have a characteristic anatomy that predisposes them to airway collapse.

177. If You Have Atrial Fibrillation, Ask If Sleep Apnea Is Causing It

If you have an irregular heart rhythm known as atrial fibrillation, ask your physician or health care provider if obstructive sleep apnea could be causing it. It is well established that untreated obstructive sleep apnea can cause or contribute to the cardiac rhythm known as atrial fibrillation. Normally, all of the chambers of the heart contract in a synchronous fashion to propel blood to all the vital organs of the body. With atrial fibrillation, two of the chambers known as the atria go into spasm. This decreases the effectiveness of the heart pumping and increases the risk of a stroke. With untreated obstructive sleep apnea, the drop in oxygen and outpouring of stimulating neurotransmitters during sleep can precipitate this spasm of the atria. Treatment of obstructive sleep apnea can eliminate this unwanted nocturnal cardiac stimulation and decrease the likelihood of a recurrence of atrial fibrillation.

178. Symptoms of Sleep Apnea Mean You Need a Sleep Study

Your physician or health care provider may order a sleep study because of a suspicion for obstructive sleep apnea. You should consider having this performed at a center accredited by the American Academy of Sleep Medicine to ensure that the study conforms to the high standards set by the Academy. Studies are typically performed at night, although daytime studies may be conducted for night shift workers.

179. Know What to Expect During a Sleep Study

During your study, expect to arrive several hours before bedtime so you have time to acclimate to the surroundings and meet with your sleep technician. Your technician will show you to your own room, typically equipped with a single bed, television, night stand, chair, closet, and sink. Bathrooms are always available and usually are right outside your room. You may share a bathroom with at least one other patient. Your technician will place monitors, including EEG (electroencephalogram), EOG (electrooculogram), and EMG (electromyogram) to determine sleep stage. EKG helps the physician monitor your cardiac rhythm. Airflow is monitored with a device that detects either temperature or pressure changes in your nose and mouth as you breathe in and out. Respiratory effort is detected by one band placed around your chest and one band placed around your abdomen. The stretch within each band transmits a signal that correlates with breathing in and out. A probe is placed on your finger to continuously monitor your blood oxygen level. Additionally, the technician will place monitors on your legs to determine whether they move during sleep. Fear not if you have a needle phobia, as many people do: No needles are used in a sleep study. The monitoring devices are painless. The timing of turning lights out can be coordinated with your normal sleep schedule, so you should inform your sleep technician of your usual bedtime. Most sleep centers will have one technician caring for two patients being studied in separate rooms. Sleep centers are commonly equipped with a total of four beds, but this varies from center to center. Typically, you will be monitored from a control room with video and audio recording. Video recording allows monitoring for abnormal movement. When you want to use the bathroom, your technician will simply detach your monitoring devices. Your sleep study will typically end six to eight hours after lights were turned out. Following your sleep study, discuss the results and treatment options with your physician. A diagnosis of obstructive sleep apnea will probably mean that you will return to the center for a second study to help you solve the problem with a device called CPAP (continuous positive airway pressure), the primary treatment for obstructive sleep apnea.

180. You Do Not Need to Sleep Soundly During Your Sleep Study

Many patients worry about the quality of sleep they have had in the sleep laboratory, and question whether the results of their study can be accurate. Sleep physicians do not expect your sleep in the laboratory to be as comfortable as at home, but nevertheless can usually obtain enough information to determine whether or not you have sleep apnea with a few hours of sleep.

181. If You Find It Hard to Relax in Unfamiliar Situations, Ask If You Can Take a Sleeping Pill to Get You Through Your Sleep Study

The goal of a sleep study is to observe you while you are asleep. If you anticipate that you will not be able to fall asleep, ask your sleep physician if you can take a sleeping pill. Sleeping pills may change your sleep architecture a bit, but several medications are available that will not have a significant impact on the frequency of sleep apnea.

182. Try to Sleep on Your Back and Your Side During Your Sleep Study

If you are able to sleep on both your back and your side, try to change positions accordingly during your study. This will give your sleep physician important information about the severity of your sleep apnea and whether or not it can be treated simply by avoiding sleeping on your back at home.

183. After Your Sleep Study, Ask about Sleep Stages and Other Findings in Addition to Changes in Breathing

Although many people undergo a sleep study to determine if they have sleep apnea, there is a wealth of additional information that you can get from the data recorded while you slept. Take a look at the tips that follow to see just what you can learn.

184. Determine Your "Sleep Efficiency"

Sleep efficiency represents the percentage of time you slept in relation to the total time you spent in bed. For example, if you were in bed for six hours but slept for only three hours, your sleep efficiency is 50 percent. As we have said, it is not surprising that people in a sleep laboratory often have low sleep efficiency, but this number will give you a sense of how well you slept.

185. Find Out Whether You Were Seen in All Sleep Stages

It is not unusual for patients in the sleep laboratory to have a reduced amount of slow-wave sleep, since they are generally not sleeping as well as they do at home. Elderly patients often have little if any slow-wave sleep. The lack of slow-wave sleep should not necessarily be a cause for concern. On the other hand, if you are being evaluated for sleep apnea, you do want to confirm that you were seen in REM sleep. Since this is the stage of sleep in which apnea is most common, a study in which no REM sleep was recorded may not provide enough information to rule out a breathing disturbance.

186. Ask If You Exhibited "Alpha-Delta" Sleep

Alpha-delta sleep, also known as "alpha intrusion in non-REM sleep" is a term that describes sleep that combines EEG features of wakefulness (alpha waves) with EEG features of non-REM sleep. Although the significance of this finding on a sleep study is unclear, some sleep physicians believe that it is an indication of un-refreshing sleep. It seems to be more common in patients with chronic pain and rheumatologic disorders, but it can be seen in patients who have no complaints.

187. Ask Whether Your Periodic Limb Movements Really Need to Be Treated

Periodic limb movements are commonly seen on sleep studies in patients who do not have any leg discomfort. We discuss in Chapter 7: Advice for People with Odd Behaviors During Sleep how periodic limb movements are a frequent companion to restless legs syndrome. But if leg movements during sleep are not bothering you or your bed partner, do not assume that they need to be treated just because they occur. Discuss whether to treat these movements with your physician; treat them only if they disrupt your sleep.

188. After Your Sleep Study, Work with Your Physician to Find an Appropriate Treatment for Your Snoring or Sleep Apnea

There are lots of options for treating snoring and sleep apnea. The most appropriate treatment for you depends on the severity of your condition. If you have sleep apnea, you may wish to look first at tips in this section that cover the use of CPAP, the most effective treatment.

189. If You Have Insomnia or an Unusual Schedule, Keep a Sleep Log Before Your Visit with a Sleep Physician

It is sometimes difficult for patients to describe their sleep patterns to a physician. If you are being evaluated for a circadian rhythm disorder or for chronic insomnia, it may be helpful for you to keep track of your sleep for several weeks before your appointment. Relevant information includes when you went to bed each night, when you woke up (during the night or in the morning) and when and how long you napped.

190. You Probably Do Not Need a Sleep Study If Your Problem Is Falling Asleep

If you see a sleep physician for help with insomnia, do not be surprised if no mention is made of obtaining a sleep study. In the majority of cases, patients with insomnia do not need to be observed in the sleep laboratory. If you have trouble falling asleep at home, you are likely to have the same trouble in the laboratory, and a sleep study during which no sleep is achieved is not productive. On the other hand, if you fall asleep easily but can't stay asleep, it may be worthwhile to monitor your sleep in order to determine what is waking you up during the night.

191. Lose Weight to Decrease Abnormal Breathing

As a first line of defense against snoring and abnormal breathing at night, lose weight if your body mass index is more than 25. A body mass index between 25 and 29.5 means you are overweight, and when it goes to 30 or more, then you are obese.

Your body mass index can be determined using the following formula:

Weight in pounds divided by
Height in inches squared
multiplied by 703
= body mass index

192. Have a Ball

Primary snoring can be treated in some surprisingly simple ways. Snoring, which is a vibration of the soft palate, can be relieved by sewing a pocket on back of your nightshirt and placing a tennis ball in that pocket. It will help keep you from sleeping on your back, which commonly provokes or worsens snoring. Another approach is to wear a fanny pack stuffed with golf balls between the shoulder blades. For some people, a more long-lasting solution, but one that requires more commitment, is weight loss. This reduces excess tissue in the airway or neck which can contribute to constriction of the breathing passage.

193. Get Checked for Nasal Obstruction

If you breathe through your mouth even when you don't have a cold, get checked for nasal obstruction. We normally breathe through our nasal passage. Chronic mouth breathing is a sure sign that the nasal passage is blocked. The cause could be allergies, a deviated septum, or swollen turbinates; correcting the latter two involves relatively minor surgery.

194. Try Nasal Strips

Try nasal strips for a few nights to see if they relieve your snoring. While these strips are probably overrated as an aid to athletic performance, they do seem to provide snoring relief for some people. According to the makers of Breathe Right strips, these adhesive bandages with a backbone help the snorer by enlarging the cross-sectional area of the nasal passages, which has the effect of increasing airflow through the nostrils.

195. Try an Oral Appliance

If your issue is mild sleep apnea, look into getting an oral appliance. Not everyone with sleep apnea needs to be treated with CPAP, a device which provides the most effective remedy (see below). An oral appliance (OA) might alleviate your problem if you are not obese and have symptoms primarily when sleeping on your back. The device does not move your jaw dramatically; it pulls the mandible forward by only 5 to 10 millimeters, which is just enough to open the airway. The tongue is attached to the mandible so the device pulls it away from the airway and that stops the snoring. Unfortunately, an OA may be costly and insurance carriers typically do not cover the cost. At the same time, it is hard to put a price on good quality sleep, so a well-fitted OA may be worth considering if your apnea is mild.

196. Make Sure the OA Fits Properly

Find a dentist or oral surgeon with lots of relevant experience to fit your OA. The use of an oral appliance can lead to side effects such as excessive salivation, dry mouth, and pain in the temporomandibular joint. It can also lead to shifts in teeth.

You want to avoid solving one problem and causing another with an OA, so make sure you go to a dentist or oral surgeon with significant experience in fitting this kind of device. And follow up with the doctor to be sure that no significant adverse effects develop.

197. Find Out about the Pillar Procedure

Ask an ear, nose and throat specialist about the Pillar Procedure. This is an outpatient procedure that can be done during an office visit. The physician inserts three small polyester implants into the soft palate. The added rigidity reduces the tendency of the structures of the soft palate to vibrate, which is what causes snoring. Make sure you discuss potential adverse effects thoroughly, since the long-term impact of this procedure is not yet known.

198. Find Out about Snoreplasty

Ask an ear, nose and throat specialist about a snoreplasty. This procedure for snoring involves injection of a stiffening agent into the soft palate. The resultant stiffening can lead to decreased vibration and, therefore, decreased snoring.

199. Ask about Radio Frequency Procedures

Ask an ear, nose and throat specialist about radio frequency procedures such as Somnoplasty and Coblation. These procedures generate heat when a probe is applied directly to the soft palate to create stiffening and decreased snoring. These procedures will likely result in pain for several days and may require a narcotic for pain relief. They are often done in the office on an outpatient basis. A successful outcome may require more than one procedure.

200. Find Out about LAUP

Ask an ear, nose and throat specialist about the LAUP. This procedure—Laser Assisted Uvula Palatoplasty—makes use of a laser to vaporize the uvula and part of the soft palate. It shortens and stiffens the soft palate to decrease snoring. The surgeon performs it after an injection of a local anesthetic similar to what a dentist uses before drilling in your tooth. Pain may be more severe than the other procedures listed above, and you will likely need a narcotic for pain control. If you choose this procedure, consider having it done on a Thursday so you can take a long weekend off from work. When you return to work on Monday, don't expect to talk a lot during the following week. You may need a second treatment three months later depending on the success of the procedure. This procedure may be considered for snoring, upper airway resistance syndrome, or mild obstructive sleep apnea, but should not be considered for more severe obstructive sleep apnea. The potential downside of this procedure is that it can eliminate snoring without eliminating the more serious associated problems of apnea.

201. Research Uvulopalatopharyngoplasty

Ask your ear, nose and throat doctor about a uvulopalatopharyngoplasty. While the LAUP described above is generally not recommended for patients with moderate or severe obstructive sleep apnea, a uvulopalatopharyngoplasty can be considered as a treatment option. If weight loss and CPAP (the treatment of choice) prove ineffective or intolerable, you may be a candidate for a uvulopalatopharyngoplasty. Seek out an experienced surgeon who performs the procedure regularly. Your sleep specialist, who often works closely with the otorhinolaryngology department (ear, nose and throat = otorhinolaryngologist) can guide you. Favorable characteristics of your airway suggesting that you will benefit from this procedure include a small tongue and large tonsils, as well as a thick long uvula and excessive tissue in the back of your throat. However, even in the hands of an experienced surgeon, there is no guarantee of a cure. Plan on having pain requiring narcotic therapy after having surgery. Plan on taking time off from work. Also plan on getting a follow up sleep study approximately three months after your surgery to assess whether the surgery has been successful and to determine whether additional therapy is necessary. Interestingly, the pain from surgery will likely contribute to decreased eating and weight loss. This, in itself, may help your obstructive sleep apnea. And after you can swallow again, try to maintain the weight loss.

202. Research Genioplasty

Ask an oral surgeon about a sliding genioplasty for your obstructive sleep apnea. This procedure involves making an incision under the lower lip. A diamond shaped incision is made to pull a fragment of bone forward several millimeters. Because the tongue is attached to this fragment of bone, it pulls the tongue forward to allow for more room in the back of the airway. This can decrease apneas by giving you a larger airway during sleep. This procedure may be suitable for patients with a small or recessed jaw. It sometimes is performed in combination with a uvulopalatopharyngoplasty. Your surgeon will let you know whether your airway appears amenable to a sliding genioplasty. Most likely, you will want to have a follow up sleep study three months after surgery to assess whether or not it has been successful and to determine if you need other therapy. There is no guarantee that this surgical procedure will lead to resolution of your obstructive sleep apnea.

203. Talk to an Oral Surgeon about the BIMAX

Maxillary-mandibular osteotomy is a surgical procedure that involves breaking both the upper and lower jaw bones. It's not nearly as bad as having it done in a street fight, though. The jaw bones are then advanced in an effort to pull the tongue forward. This increases the airway space during sleep and can result in resolution of obstructive sleep apnea. This is aggressive surgery that is generally only considered in patients who find other surgical and non-surgical interventions unsuccessful. This procedure should be performed by a very experienced surgeon, typically at a regional specialized center.

204. If All Else Fails, You May Need a Tracheostomy

Although a relatively extreme measure, a tracheostomy may save your life. For patients who have severe obstructive sleep apnea with life threatening problems such as severe coronary disease, dangerous cardiac arrhythmias or congestive heart failure, a tracheostomy may be considered if previously outlined measures have been unsuccessful. This surgery involves making an incision in your windpipe and placing a curved tube that sits in your windpipe. As you breathe through this opening during sleep, you bypass the obstruction higher up behind your tongue and soft palate. A cap can be placed on the tube to allow for normal speech and breathing during the day.

205. Ask Your Doctor about a Tonsillectomy

Even adults can benefit from tonsillectomy for treatment of obstructive sleep apnea. While children with obstructive sleep apnea frequently benefit from tonsillectomy, adults may benefit as well. In the non obese-patient with very large tonsils and obstructive sleep apnea, tonsillectomy is often beneficial. Many people make it to adulthood with tonsils intact. Most can stay that way. However, if you have frequent infections of the tonsils, known as tonsillitis, or if you have loud snoring, upper airway resistance syndrome, or obstructive sleep apnea, you will likely benefit from having your very large tonsils removed. Tonsillectomy is usually painful and will require likely narcotic therapy as well as some time off from work. While sometimes performed on an outpatient basis, your surgeon will want to consider a night's stay in the hospital for close monitoring if you have obstructive sleep apnea. The overweight or obese patient with large tonsils and obstructive sleep apnea may benefit from a trial of weight loss and CPAP prior to tonsillectomy. Following weight loss, symptoms of obstructive sleep apnea may improve even without removal of the tonsils. This, in part, will likely depend on how large your tonsils are. If they are "kissing" tonsils, almost completely obstructing your airway, then removal will likely prove beneficial for the overweight or obese patient as well.

206. Get the Right Surgeon to Perform Your Snore-Aid Procedures

When choosing a physician to perform any procedure designed to treat sleep-disordered breathing, ask the following questions:

- How much will the procedure cost? Note that insurance companies typically will not cover procedures for snoring in the absence of apneas.
- How many sessions will be necessary to eliminate snoring?
- Will I need narcotics for pain control?
- How much time will I need to take off from work?
- How often do you do this procedure and how many procedures have you performed? If the physician performs this procedure less than once a month, consider finding someone with more experience.
- Have any of your patients developed complications from this procedure?
- What is your success rate with this procedure?

207. Don't Hesitate to Try a Nasal CPAP Machine

A nasal CPAP machine is the treatment of choice for obstructive sleep apnea. The nasal passages are connected to the back of the throat and this simple anatomical fact underlies the reason why CPAP—Continuous Positive Airway Pressure—is so effective. This portable device, invented by C.E. Sullivan in 1982, includes a blower unit typically the size of a half loaf of bread, tubing, and an interface that attaches to your nose, or covers your nose and mouth. The air acts as a splint to keep the airway from collapsing when you sleep. The amount of air coming in depends on your particular need.

208. Identify the CPAP Mask or Facial Attachment That You Find Most Comfortable

Since the invention of CPAP, many improvements have been made to increase the comfort of the interface. Three different types of interfaces can be used, depending on your preference. These options include soft prongs, or pillows, that rest in the nose, a nasal mask that covers the nose, or a full face mask over the nose and mouth. If you have obstructive sleep apnea, you should spend time with the sleep staff in your sleep center to determine which interface feels most comfortable for you. It is not uncommon for patients to switch interfaces over time, based on comfort. Wear and tear of the CPAP interface may lead you to request a new one as often as every six months. Typically, insurance carriers will cover this expense, in addition to the blower unit and tubing. For many people, it may take a period of days to weeks to get used to it, so if you find it annoying at first, persevere, but let your doctor know that you are having a challenging time so you can find solutions to the problem together. The benefits of the therapy are well worth the effort.

209. Add Humidity to the Process If You Have Nasal Stuffiness When Using CPAP

Airway dryness is often minimized with the use of a heated humidifier built directly into the blower unit. Most people now advocate routinely using heated humidification to decrease nasal symptoms. If symptoms persist despite use of a heated humidifier, nasal sprays such as a nasal steroid or saline may relieve symptoms. Over-the-counter saline sprays are readily available.

210. Lower the CPAP Pressure

Ask your physician to try a lower CPAP pressure if the current one seems too strong. The average CPAP pressure to maintain an open airway for a patient with obstructive sleep apnea is between 7 and 11 cm of water pressure. Some patients require as much as 20 cm of water pressure. If your pressure feels too strong and you feel you cannot tolerate it, a lower pressure, while not perfect, may be more tolerable. It makes no sense to keep you on a high pressure that you cannot use on a regular basis. A lower CPAP pressure may not eliminate all of your snoring and apneas, but it likely will be better than no CPAP at all. After you have gotten used to the sensation of CPAP, you may be able to tolerate a higher pressure.

211. Try Adaptive Servo-Ventilation

If CPAP seems to have worsened your sleep apnea, adaptive servo-ventilation may be the answer. CPAP is a remarkably effective treatment for most patients with sleep apnea. A few patients, however, find that their pattern of breathing becomes more irregular on CPAP. They may develop "central" sleep apneas: pauses in breathing which are not caused by obstruction. A new technology called adaptive servo-ventilation (ASV) can be very helpful in this situation. ASV provides a variable pressure when you inhale, and a fixed pressure when you exhale. Establishing the correct settings for an ASV unit will require an additional sleep study, but the improvement in breathing at night may be dramatic.

212. Be Honest about the Amount of Time You Use CPAP

A number of studies have shown that patients with sleep apnea overestimate the number of nights and hours that they use CPAP. CPAP is effective only if you use it, not if it sits unused on the nightstand. Most of the new CPAP machines contain monitoring technology which allows you and your doctor to assess your days and hours of CPAP use. This technology also monitors mask leaks and estimates the number of apneas that are still occurring. If you are being started on CPAP, ask to be outfitted with a CPAP machine that has this capability.

213. Bring Your CPAP with You on Your Vacation

While you may be tempted to leave your CPAP at home, don't. Treatment of obstructive sleep apnea requires regular nightly use. If you skip it while you are on vacation, your apneas and the cardiovascular stress it causes will recur. Also, why feel lousy on your vacation? Don't check in your CPAP machine with your suitcases. It is a delicate piece of equipment that should be hand carried with you onto the airplane. Most airport security guards are familiar with CPAP devices.

214. Try Bilevel Pressure

Really hate CPAP? Try bilevel pressure. Some people find nasal CPAP intolerable during exhalation only. If you have tried to adjust to CPAP, but have difficulty exhaling, then an alternative that may work for you is Bilevel Positive Airway Pressure. This modality is also sometimes used if you have COPD (chronic obstructive pulmonary disease). With bilevel pressure, the pressure during exhalation is significantly decreased. You may find this more tolerable. While there is no evidence that bilevel pressure is better than CPAP for obstructive sleep apnea syndrome, it may be necessary for you to tolerate positive airway pressure. Switching to bilevel pressure will likely require an additional night in the sleep center for a repeat titration to determine optimal pressure settings.

215. Try APAP

Restless sleeper with CPAP? Try APAP. For patients requiring very high pressures of nasal CPAP, a newer device known as APAP, or Autoadjusting Positive Airway Pressure may decrease the average pressure during the night. This device will adjust by itself during sleep when you stop breathing to provide adequate airflow. The pressure required may change depending on position and the stage of sleep. For example, when you are on your back in REM sleep, it is likely that the pressure requirement will be high. When you are in non-REM sleep on your side, a lower pressure may relieve obstruction completely. So, if you are having difficulty tolerating your high CPAP pressure, ask about APAP.

216. Prior to Surgery, Tell Your Doctor If You Have Sleep Apnea

The effects of anesthesia and postoperative narcotics and sedatives can be deadly for patients with obstructive sleep apnea. These medications can have a relaxing effect on the airway leading to worsening apnea and a more severe drop in oxygen levels. This can lead to an unexpected stroke, heart attack, or cardiopulmonary arrest resulting in neurological injury or death. If general anesthesia is planned, an overnight stay with careful monitoring and avoidance of over-sedation is often recommended. You will want to wear your CPAP each night while in the hospital.

217. If You Have Severe Obstructive Sleep Apnea, Find Out If You Need a Pacemaker

On rare occasions, people with obstructive sleep apnea need a pacemaker. In some patients with obstructive sleep apnea, the heart stops during sleep for more than five seconds. It resumes when the apnea ends. Treatment with CPAP is usually all that is necessary. However, for more prolonged periods of heart block, a pacemaker should be considered. This will require discussion between you, your sleep physician, and a cardiologist.

218. Take Your CPAP to the Hospital If You're Admitted

If you have obstructive sleep apnea and regularly use CPAP, you will want to bring your unit with you for nightly use. Your hospital may have rules requiring the use of its own equipment. However, ask if you can bring your own machine because you have become accustomed to it. If this is not allowed, at least bring in your CPAP mask and inform your health care provider of your CPAP pressure setting. You certainly will want to continue effective therapy of your obstructive sleep apnea during your hospital stay.

219. Get an Echocardiogram After Your Sleep Apnea Is Treated

If you have congestive heart failure, get an echocardiogram after your obstructive sleep apnea is treated. Many patients with congestive heart failure also have obstructive sleep apnea. Nocturnal hypoxia and catecholamine release from the adrenal glands due to frequent apneas during sleep can worsen cardiac function. However, with treatment of obstructive sleep apnea, cardiac function can improve significantly. One such measure of cardiac function is the echocardiogram. With use of an ultrasound, the echocardiogram can determine the ejection fraction of your heart. The ejection fraction tells us the percentage of blood that is ejected from the heart chambers with each cardiac contraction. A low ejection fraction is a sign of a failing heart. The ejection fraction may improve significantly following treatment of your obstructive sleep apnea. This can lead to decreased symptoms associated with congestive heart failure, as well as a decreased need for medical therapy. On rare occasions, a patient listed for cardiac transplant may no longer require this surgical intervention after obstructive sleep apnea is treated.

220. Get Checked for Cushing's Syndrome

If you have unexpectedly gained weight, developed a round moon-shaped face, diabetes, and high blood pressure, then get checked for Cushing's syndrome. Cushing's syndrome can result from a tumor in your pituitary or adrenal gland, resulting in overproduction of the hormone cortisol. This condition can also result from the ingestion of systemic steroids used for various medical conditions such as asthma or arthritis. With weight gain and narrowing of the airway in the back of your throat, obstructive sleep apnea can develop. The diagnosis can be established with blood and urine testing. Treatment may require surgery to remove the tumor making too much hormone, or a decrease in systemic steroids that are used to treat your inflammatory condition.

221. Get Checked for Acromegaly

If rings and shoes no longer fit, and your jaw looks bigger, get checked for acromegaly. The pituitary is a very small gland in your brain that is responsible for the production of many hormones that regulate various functions in the body. One such hormone is responsible for growth. A small tumor in the pituitary gland can produce too much growth hormone that can cause your jaw, nose, feet, and hands to get bigger. Your tongue might also become enlarged, which would cause or contribute to obstructive sleep apnea. A diagnosis of acromegaly can easily be made with blood testing. Often, the treatment is microsurgery to remove the tumor, after which you should see a reduction in all the symptoms, including obstructive sleep apnea.

222. Get Checked for Polycythemia

If your physician tells you that you have polycythemia, consider the possibility of obstructive sleep apnea. Polycythemia is a condition where you have too many red blood cells in your bloodstream. Red blood cells circulate in your bloodstream to deliver oxygen to your cells. If you have too few red blood cells, you are anemic. If you have too many, you have polycythemia. This disorder can result from low oxygen levels during sleep. This leads to an increased production of the chemical called erythropoietin. Erythropoietin stimulates your bone marrow to produce more red blood cells. An excess of red blood cells in your bloodstream raises the concern of a primary bone marrow problem or a secondary problem such as insufficient oxygen during sleep. This, in combination with snoring or other symptoms of obstructive sleep apnea should lead to obtaining a sleep study.

223. Ask Your Physician about Obstructive Sleep Apnea as a Cause of Protein in Your Urine

If your physician tells you that you have protein in your urine specimen, consider the possibility of obstructive sleep apnea. While the exact cause is unclear, patients with obstructive sleep apnea can develop protein in the urine. If you snore, or have other symptoms suggestive of obstructive sleep apnea, and have protein in your urine, a sleep study should be considered.

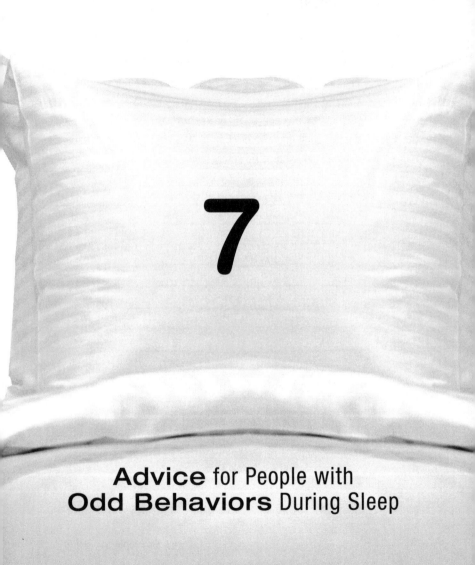

7

Advice for People with
Odd Behaviors During Sleep

224. Get a Family Sleep History Before Seeing Your Sleep Physician

225. Enjoy the Mumbling

226. In General, Don't Worry about Twitching or Jerking

227. Get Checked for Propriospinal Myoclonus

228. Understand the Nature of Sleepwalking

229. If You Have a History of Sleepwalking, Be Cautious about the Use of Sleeping Pills

230. You May Not Need to Be Treated for Confusional Arousals

231. Discuss Your Sleep Patterns with Your Physician If There Is Evidence That You Are Leaving the Bed or Bedroom While Asleep

232. Tell Your Partner to Sit Tight If You Have a Night Terror

233. Seek Evaluation If You Commonly Experience Sleepwalking or Night Terrors as an Adult

234. Avoid Alcohol, Stress, and Sleep Deprivation If You Sleepwalk

235. Hide Car Keys and Secure the Environment If You Sleepwalk

236. Don't Wake a Sleepwalker

237. See a Sleep Physician If You Exhibit Odd Behaviors at Night

238. Identify the Cause of Nocturnal Eating

239. Seek Treatment If You Are a Night-Eater

255. Beware of Augmentation

256. If You Have RLS, Forgo Donating Blood on a Regular Basis

257. Don't Confuse Leg Cramps with RLS

258. If You Have RLS, Alert Your Bed Partner

259. Rock Yourself to Sleep

260. Identify the Cause of Nighttime Headaches

261. Seek Evaluation and Treatment for Cluster Headaches

262. If You Develop Headaches Late in Life, Seek Evaluation

263. If You Suffer from Migraines, Sleep Can Be Friend or Foe

264. Ask Your Dentist If You Suffer from Bruxism

265. Wear a Bite Guard

266. Change Your Body Position

The word "parasomnia" refers to any undesirable event or behavior that occurs during sleep. We cover common parasomnias in this chapter, as well as a few uncommon ones. Childhood parasomnias are also discussed in Chapter 5, which provides advice to individuals with children. Some parasomnias are considered normal events—most notably sleepwalking and talking in your sleep—although they may be disturbing to those who experience them or to family members.

224. Get a Family Sleep History Before Seeing Your Sleep Physician

Knowing your family history will help you get a good night's sleep. If you are being evaluated for a sleep disorder, ask your close relatives if they have any sleep difficulties. Sleep disorders that may run in families include restless legs syndrome, sleepwalking, and advanced or delayed sleep phase. Relatives of patients with narcolepsy have a somewhat increased risk of this disorder. It is not unusual for several members of the same family to have sleep apnea.

225. Enjoy the Mumbling

Talking in sleep is normal for many people. Sleep talking (somniloquy) can occur in any stage of sleep. The content of speech during sleep is variable: Occasionally people utter complete phrases or sentences, at other times they just moan or mumble.

226. In General, Don't Worry about Twitching or Jerking

Most of us have occasionally been aware of suddenly jerking or twitching as we fall asleep. If these body jerks are brief and occur only as we fall asleep, they are called sleep starts or hypnic jerks. Less common than hypnic jerks are other unusual sensations at the transition between wakefulness and sleep. These sensations are referred to as sensory sleep starts, and they may consist of the illusion of falling, or the illusion of a sudden loud noise or flash of light. A severe form of sensory sleep starts has been called "the exploding head syndrome"; this particular sensation, as its name suggests, can be distressing, but like other sleep starts, it is benign and does not require treatment.

227. Get Checked for Propriospinal Myoclonus

If sudden movement as you begin to relax prevents you from falling asleep, you may need medication to treat it. You might have a condition called propriospinal myoclonus. These sudden jerking, twisting, or bending movements of the neck and trunk can occur when you are in relaxed wakefulness and interfere with your ability to fall asleep. Unlike sleep starts, which arise in drowsiness, propiospinal myoclonus happens when you are still awake. It's rare, but can be disturbing to those who experience it. It can be treated with medication.

228. Understand the Nature of Sleepwalking

In sleepwalking, you are awake and asleep simultaneously. Although typically the brain cycles in a controlled fashion between wakefulness and the various stages of sleep, situations can arise in which the boundaries between wakefulness and sleep become blurred. When this occurs, you can exhibit a variety of unusual behaviors. These behaviors include confusional arousals, sleepwalking, and night terrors. These particular behaviors are referred to as "disorders of arousal," and they share several features: They are common in children, they tend to run in families, and they tend to occur in the first third of the night, when partial wakefulness intrudes into deep (slow-wave) sleep. Typically, you will have minimal or no recall of the episode the following day.

229. If You Have a History of Sleepwalking, Be Cautious about the Use of Sleeping Pills

Sleepwalking has been reported with the use of certain sleeping pills. Make sure you discuss the choice of sleeping pills with your doctor if you need medication for insomnia.

230. You May Not Need to Be Treated for Confusional Arousals

If your bed partner notices brief awakenings that you do not remember, you may be having confusional arousals. Confusional arousals are short-lasting apparent awakenings in which you will seem momentarily startled or confused, and then you will go back to sleep. When individuals do have recall of these events, they may wish to be treated, but otherwise this is usually unnecessary.

231. Discuss Your Sleep Patterns with Your Physician If There Is Evidence That You Are Leaving the Bed or Bedroom While Asleep

The activity of some sleepwalkers is more elaborate than just walking. Not only do they appear to awaken, but they leave the bed and can leave the bedroom, and they can sometimes perform complex tasks such as moving furniture or eating, without actually waking up.

232. Tell Your Partner to Sit Tight If You Have a Night Terror

A night terror is the most dramatic disorder of arousal. When night terrors occur, you will not only appear to be awake, but also seem profoundly frightened, with dilated pupils, sweating and a rapid heartbeat. Night terrors often begin with a scream. The episodes may last for several minutes. Attempts to flee from the imagined threat may occur. Yet in spite of the apparent violence of these episodes, you won't recall them in the morning. There is little that a bed partner can do to terminate an episode of night terrors, but a sleep physician should be consulted to determine if preventive treatment is necessary.

233. Seek Evaluation If You Commonly Experience Sleepwalking or Night Terrors as an Adult

Children commonly experience confusional arousals, sleepwalking, and night terrors, but seek evaluation if you have them as an adult. A small percentage of individuals with a childhood history of sleepwalking or related disorder continue to exhibit the same behavior as adults. Such adults may be suspected of having a psychiatric disturbance, but generally this is not the case. Like childhood sleepwalkers, these adults do not have well-defined sleep stages, and they may at times be in a "dissociated" or mixed state of wakefulness and sleep. If you have sleepwalking or night terrors as an adult, you should be evaluated and treated at a sleep center.

234. Avoid Alcohol, Stress, and Sleep Deprivation If You Sleepwalk

If you have a history of sleepwalking, avoid the precipitating factors of alcohol and sleep deprivation. If you take a sleeping medication, ask your doctor if reports indicate it may be linked to sleepwalking.

235. Hide Car Keys and Secure the Environment If You Sleepwalk

Sleepwalkers have been known to get in a car and drive, go to the kitchen and cook, and even attack others. They don't remember it and don't know why they did it. Although it's extremely rare that a sleepwalker will take action like this, if you know you have ever walked in your sleep, take a few extra precautions so you don't put yourself or others in harm's way.

236. Don't Wake a Sleepwalker

You should not try to wake up a sleepwalker. Sleepwalkers may become confused, irritable, or even violent if you try to awaken them. Since sleepwalkers are "caught" in a state in which they are neither fully awake nor fully asleep, their response to interference from others may be unpredictable. It is appropriate simply to guide sleepwalkers gently back to bed, and to secure the environment to ensure that they do not wander into situations that may be dangerous.

237. See a Sleep Physician If You Exhibit Odd Behaviors at Night

If you are exhibiting odd behaviors at night, you should be evaluated by a sleep specialist. The decision to medically treat nocturnal behaviors should be made on an individualized basis. Sleepwalking in children may not require treatment. Establishing a safe environment and reassuring parents that sleepwalking is likely to disappear over time may be all that is necessary. However, in patients, whether children or adults, who appear to be at high risk of injury, evaluation in a sleep center is recommended. A sleep center evaluation is particularly important in identifying the cause of the sleep disturbance. Patients who believe that they are sleepwalking may in fact be having nocturnal seizures or displaying symptoms of REM sleep behavior disorder (see the next entries). These disorders have entirely different implications and treatment requirements.

238. Identify the Cause of Nocturnal Eating

Eating at night can take several forms. Some people eat during the night with complete awareness as a self-soothing mechanism. Some nighttime eaters, including those with an eating disorder, may be consuming calories at night that they deny themselves during the day. But when eating occurs without awareness and without recall, that's "sleep-related eating disorder." This is analogous to other seemingly purposeful behaviors that can occur during sleep. Sometimes the only evidence of sleep-related eating is crumbs in the bedroom or dishes in the kitchen in the morning. Sometimes, people with this problem try to eat plants, paper, and other non-food items.

239. Seek Treatment If You Are a Night-Eater

If you are a night-eater, seek medical evaluation. A variety of behavioral techniques and medications can be used to treat night-eating, depending on the cause.

240. Don't Be Embarrassed to Talk to Your Doctor about Sleep-Related Sexual Behavior

Sexual behavior during sleep is a recently described parasomnia. If we can talk, walk, and eat during sleep without awareness, it is not surprising that other behaviors can occur as well. In the last several years there have been a number of descriptions in the medical literature of people who engage in sexual activity during sleep, including masturbation and uninvited sexual advances toward bed partners. This can be disruptive to a relationship. If you have had such experiences, you may wish to seek treatment at a sleep center.

241. Seek Evaluation If Your Dreams Have Changed

Nightmares are a universal experience, but seek evaluation if there is a change in the frequency or pattern of your dreams. The typical nightmare awakens you from sleep and you may be able to remember full details of what has frightened you, or simply fragments and images. Nightmares are common in children, but can occur in adults as well, often during a period of stress. Although they're unpleasant, nightmares should not cause you alarm. When should you be worried about your bad dreams? If they become unusually frequent, or if the content consists of "flashbacks" to a traumatic experience, you may have an underlying mood disorder or post-traumatic stress disorder and should discuss this change in the pattern of dreaming with your physician.

242. Speak to a Doctor If You Act Out Your Dreams

You may have REM Sleep Behavior Disorder, which puts you at risk of injuring yourself or someone else. Normally when you are in REM sleep (the stage in which most dreaming occurs), you have a very limited ability to move your arms and legs. Your muscles may twitch briefly, and you may be able to talk or call out, but you should not be able to perform any complicated actions. If you were able to run, punch, jump, or kick as the imaginary events in your dreams unfolded, you would place yourself and your bed partner at risk of injury. This is exactly what happens when people develop REM Sleep Behavior Disorder (RBD), a condition in which the normal paralysis of arms and legs in REM sleep is lost. Before RBD was identified as a specific and treatable sleep disorder, patients would devise elaborate ways to restrain themselves during sleep, place padding on the floor next to their bed, or sleep apart from their partners. Now most patients can be effectively treated with clonazepam, a medication taken at bedtime that eliminates the episodes of dream enactment.

243. If You Act Out Your Dreams, You Should Be Evaluated for Neurologic Problems

RBD most often develops in men in their fifties and sixties. Unfortunately, as many as half these patients may develop Parkinson's disease or a similar neurologic illness, and so if you are treated for this disorder, you should be followed by a neurologist.

244. Make Your Bedroom a Safe Place

If you have symptoms suggestive of REM Sleep Behavior Disorder, consider placing your mattress on the floor and remove sharp objects until effective treatment has been instituted.

245. Don't Worry about Sleep Paralysis

If you awaken and are momentarily unable to move, stay calm. Give yourself a few extra seconds to wake up. You may be experiencing sleep paralysis. Like REM Sleep Behavior Disorder, sleep paralysis is due to a glitch in the control of muscle activity during REM sleep. As mentioned above, muscle activity is normally inhibited in REM sleep. If the ability to move is preserved, dream enactment can occur. If, on the other hand, the inhibition of muscle activity is not perfectly synchronized with the termination of REM sleep, muscle paralysis may continue briefly after awakening.

246. Don't Worry about Suffocation During Sleep Paralysis

When sleep paralysis occurs, it may be frightening, and sometimes there is a sense of suffocation. Fortunately, breathing is not actually compromised. Sleep paralysis typically lasts for seconds only. Many people experience it a few times over the course of their lives. It is much more common in patients with narcolepsy who may have such episodes not only when they awaken from REM sleep, but also immediately upon falling asleep. Rarely, individuals who do not have narcolepsy can have frequent episodes of sleep paralysis as well.

247. Describe Sleep-Related Movements to Your Physician

Some sleep-related movements are voluntary and others are not under conscious control. Movements that occur during the transition from wakefulness to sleep or during sleep itself are called sleep-related movement disorders. Distinguishing between voluntary and involuntary movements is helpful in establishing the diagnosis of the specific movement disorder. Several common sleep-related movement disorders are discussed in the following tips.

248. Check to See If You Have Restless Legs Syndrome

If you have an urge to move your legs as you try to fall asleep, use this checklist to see if you might have RLS. Restless Legs Syndrome (RLS) has four major characteristics.

1. Individuals with RLS have uncomfortable sensations in their legs that produce an urge to move. These sensations can be described as tingling, crawling, or painful. Many people with RLS find the sensation hard to describe.
2. Regardless of how the discomfort is experienced, movement of the legs provides temporary relief.
3. The leg symptoms are typically worse at rest, particularly when lying down or in a confined space such as a car or theater seat.
4. The symptoms typically have a circadian pattern. They tend to be worse in the evening and at bedtime.

249. If You Have RLS, Make Sure You are Not Iron Deficient

RLS is sometimes a symptom of iron deficiency. If you have symptoms of RLS that began in childhood, you are likely to have a family history of RLS, and it probably does not indicate the presence of any other medical disorder. In contrast, if you developed RLS in adulthood, you should be evaluated for iron deficiency.

250. If You Have RLS and are Pregnant, You Might Need More Iron

RLS is common in pregnancy. If RLS develops during pregnancy, it may mean you need more than what's in your prenatal vitamins. Both iron deficiency and folate deficiency occur during pregnancy. Typical prenatal vitamins may not be adequate to treat these conditions. If iron and/or folate deficiencies are the culprit, then treatment may lead to quick improvement. Avoiding alcohol and nicotine is appropriate in pregnancy and in some individuals may also help to reduce RLS. Massage therapy and warm baths may also prove beneficial.

251. Alert a Doctor to Your RLS If You Have Advanced Kidney Disease

RLS is common in patients with chronic renal failure, especially in dialysis patients. Certain medications may be helpful in the setting of kidney disease and others should be avoided. Discuss the management of this symptom with your nephrologist.

252. Be Aware of Medications That Can Worsen Your RLS Symptoms

Some antidepressants and other psychiatric medications can make RLS worse. If you need an antidepressant and suffer from RLS, buproprion may be the best choice. Over-the-counter antihistamines and caffeine can also exacerbate RLS.

253. Seek Medical Treatment for RLS

A number of drugs can be effective in treating RLS. Commonly used drugs include dopamine agonists, which mimic the action of the neurotransmitter dopamine, mild opiates such as codeine or propoxyphene, gabapentin (an anti-seizure medication), and clonazepam. Iron replacement can be helpful when patients are iron-deficient or when the serum ferritin level (another marker of the availability of iron) is less than 50 mg/ml. Vitamin C can assist with iron absorption. Among the drugs listed above, only the dopamine agonists pramipexole (Mirapex) and ropinirole (Requip) are approved by the Food and Drug Administration for the treatment of RLS.

254. Beware of Side Effects with the Most Commonly Used Drugs to Treat RLS

Potential side effects of the dopamine agonists (pramipexole and ropinirole) include nausea, lightheadedness, and rarely sleepiness or confusion. These side effects are more common in the elderly and are seldom encountered at the doses used to treat RLS. Although the dopamine agonists were developed to treat Parkinson's disease, there is no evidence that patients with RLS are at risk of this disorder.

255. Beware of Augmentation

High doses of dopamine agonists used to treat RLS can actually worsen this disorder. If that happens, discuss the problem with the doctor who prescribed the medication. Ironically, ropinirole, pramipexole and carbidopa/levodopa (Sinemet), all effective treatments for RLS, can sometimes cause symptoms to occur earlier in the day, and spread to other limbs. This is called "augmentation." If augmentation occurs, speak to your health care provider about discontinuing the offending drug, at least temporarily, and find an alternative until the symptoms improve.

256. If You Have RLS, Forgo Donating Blood on a Regular Basis

Blood donation may temporarily worsen your symptoms. Because of the association between iron deficiency anemia and RLS, patients with RLS should avoid frequent blood donation.

257. Don't Confuse Leg Cramps with RLS

There are a number of other causes of leg discomfort that can be confused with RLS. One of the most common is leg cramps. If you have a leg cramp or "charley horse," you will have a muscle spasm (often in the calf) that you can see or feel. RLS does not involve any involuntary contraction of muscles. Nocturnal leg cramps have a variety of causes, including low potassium levels. They may respond to quinine or tonic water. If you wish to treat leg cramps, you should have routine blood work to make certain that your electrolytes are normal, and then talk with your physician to be certain that quinine is safe for you.

258. If You Have RLS, Alert Your Bed Partner

Your RLS may cause you to kick during sleep. The majority of patients with RLS exhibit repetitive twitching of the legs during sleep, called Periodic Limb Movements. These twitching movements, called "periodic" because they occur at regular intervals, generally occur in the lighter stages of sleep. The twitches typically occur every twenty to forty seconds and may involve one or both legs. Occasionally, the arms may twitch at regular intervals as well. Many people with periodic limb movements are unaware of these twitches and they are brought to attention by the bed partner. Although most patients with RLS have periodic limb movements, most patients with periodic limb movements do not have RLS, and do not require treatment. Periodic limb movements are very common in the elderly. If the leg or limb movements seem to be disrupting sleep, they can be treated with the same drugs that are used to treat RLS.

259. Rock Yourself to Sleep

Go ahead and rock yourself to sleep—gently. Rocking movements of a cradle or the gentle vibrations of a car in motion tend to put children to sleep. Some children develop their own self-soothing movements to induce sleep. These efforts at self-soothing may take the form of extreme rhythmic movement, including repetitive headbanging on a wall, crib side, or mattress. These more violent rhythmic movements at sleep onset rarely persist into adulthood—but they can. They are more likely to be seen in adults with developmental disabilities, but are not limited to this group.

260. Identify the Cause of Nighttime Headaches

While the majority of headaches develop when we are awake, some headaches have a specific relationship to sleep. Headaches can be a symptom of disrupted breathing during sleep. If you snore loudly, are sleepy during the daytime and awaken with headaches, you should be evaluated for obstructive sleep apnea.

261. Seek Evaluation and Treatment for Cluster Headaches

If your headache happens around the same time every night, get checked for cluster headaches. Cluster headaches, relatively brief but severe headaches often associated with tearing and a runny nose, are a particularly painful form of headache, which primarily affects young men. The pain of cluster headaches is unilateral and is experienced in or around the eye. Cluster headaches, as their name suggests, tend to occur in series, interrupting sleep at the same time each night for several weeks in a row. They can occur in the daytime as well. If you suffer from cluster headaches, go to a neurologist.

262. If You Develop Headaches Late in Life, Seek Evaluation

Elderly men may develop severe headaches during sleep. These headaches, called "hypnic headaches," are relatively brief, lasting up to one hour. They can occur during naps as well as during nocturnal sleep. Other causes of headache need to be considered as well. Any new onset headaches or change in headache pattern should be evaluated by a physician.

263. If You Suffer from Migraines, Sleep Can Be Friend or Foe

Migraine headaches can develop during sleep. They may in particular arise from REM sleep, although the reason for this is unknown. Ironically, while some patients awaken with migraines, sleep provides relief to most patients who experience them.

264. Ask Your Dentist If You Suffer from Bruxism

A headache and a toothache mean it is time to talk to your dentist. The technical term for teeth-grinding or clenching your teeth during sleep is bruxism. It is a common disorder, particularly for people under a lot of stress. You may identify it yourself by waking up with a sore jaw, but often bed partners or other household members notice the grinding sound, or dentists notice excessive wear on your teeth during routine exams. You may even grind yourself awake. In addition to tooth wear, bruxism can also aggravate temporo-mandibular joint syndrome (TMJ).

265. Wear a Bite Guard

Wear a bite guard every night to stop grinding your teeth in your sleep. If you have bruxism you can either have a dentist custom-make a bite guard for you, or try one of the off-the-shelf brands. Muscle relaxants are also used to treat bruxism. Bruxism is not necessarily a life-long problem, and it may improve spontaneously, particularly after stressors have resolved.

266. Change Your Body Position

Do you have a mild headache or neck pain? Try changing your body position. If you awaken with headaches or neck pain, consider whether you may be sleeping in an uncomfortable position. Sometimes a change in head elevation or pillow type can alleviate headaches.

8

Advice for People with Medical Conditions

298. If You Have Parkinson's Disease, Discuss Sleep Problems with Your Neurologist

299. Seek Help If You Are Having Difficulty Caring for a Relative with Alzheimer's Disease Who Is "Sundowning"

300. Try a Bilevel Pressure Unit If You Have a Nerve or Muscle Disorder Causing Weakness

301. Look into Therapy If You Have PTSD

302. Get Help for Depression

303. Get Checked for an Ulcer

304. You May Need a Ventilator If You Have a Spinal Cord Injury

305. If You Had Polio, Get Evaluated for Sleep-Related Breathing Problems

306. Get Checked for Hyperthyroidism

307. Find Out the Source of Nocturnal Choking

Starting with acid reflux, which affects an estimated 5 to 7 percent of the population worldwide, and likely twice that percentage in the United States alone, this chapter covers a spectrum of conditions that can profoundly affect a good night's sleep. The recommendations include ways to mitigate the effects of the condition as it relates to sleep as well as signs that you need to recognize to help you prevent a potentially life threatening problem from developing.

ACID REFLUX

267. Clean Up Your Diet

Minimize the possibility of reflux by cleaning up your diet. Even if you don't eat during the four hours before bedtime as prescribed in an earlier chapter, ingestion of fatty, fried meals can contribute to reflux. Choose a low-fat, non-fried meal for dinner.

268. Have Your Main Meal Midday

If you suffer from reflux at night, consider moving your larger meal to midday. The many hours of upright posture that follow will decrease the chance of reflux at night. Have a smaller meal at the traditional dinnertime.

269. Avoid Acidic Fruits and Vegetables in the Evening

That delicious glass of orange juice or large cup of freshly cut pineapple should be avoided at dinner time. The acidic content will magnify reflux problems as you are supine in bed and ready for sleep.

270. Avoid the Mint

Resist the urge to grab a mint when leaving a restaurant. That neatly wrapped peppermint comes at a cost. It can contribute to heartburn and sleep disruption.

271. Pass on the Late-Night Candy Bar

Not only does chocolate contain the stimulant caffeine, it can, for many, contribute to reflux. Have your sweets earlier in the day and, of course, in moderation.

272. Avoid Alcohol at Night

Here's one more reason to avoid alcohol at night. In addition to the sleep disruption that alcohol causes, it can contribute to problems with reflux.

273. Avoid Caffeine at Night

Another reason to avoid caffeine. Coffee, tea, or soda containing caffeine can contribute to reflux in addition to the stimulating effects as previously described.

274. See Your Doctor about Your Heartburn

See your physician if all of the above measures are inadequate and you still wake up with heartburn. Your physician will want to make sure that you are not having a more serious problem such as heart disease.

275. Consider Medications for Reflux

Once your physician has determined that your nocturnal awakening is from reflux and not a heart problem, medical therapy may be necessary. If the above more conservative measures are unsuccessful, widely used medications, including H2 blockers such as Zantac (ranitidine) and proton pump inhibitors such as Prilosec (omeprazole) or Nexium (esomeprazole), may be extremely helpful.

276. Watch Your Use of Over-the-Counter Antacids

Occasional use of an over-the-counter antacid can provide quick relief for that unexpected episode of heartburn at nighttime. However, over reliance and daily use suggest a problem that requires more aggressive evaluation and treatment. If you are reaching for the antacid bottle more than two or three times a week, see your physician for further advice.

277. Look Into Surgery

Take a look at surgical therapy if all else fails. Occasionally, severe refractory reflux may require surgical intervention. Even if you have tried all of the above measures, you may be one of the few who continues to have sleep disruption from acid entering into the esophagus and possibly the lungs. This may be due to a faulty sphincter between the esophagus and the stomach. Normally, the lower esophageal sphincter has a thin piece of muscle that closes shut after food enters into the stomach. If the sphincter isn't working properly, a procedure known as a Nissen fundoplication can be performed with small incisions through laparoscopic surgery in the abdomen. Tightening of this sphincter muscle can prevent subsequent reflux from occurring.

278. Elevate Your Head

To avoid nocturnal gastro-esophageal reflux disease (GERD) symptoms, elevate the head of your bed with bricks about six inches high. About ten percent of the population has a hiatal hernia, or opening in the diaphragm that allows part of the stomach to slip up into the chest. This condition predisposes the sufferer toward reflux, regardless of when or what the person eats. Pillows will not create the angle needed to avert the problem. You need to increase the incline of the stomach and the esophagus (food pipe.) Elevate the whole head of the bed by slipping a brick under each bedpost at the head. Most gastroenterologists suggest 6" of elevation.

279. If You're Asthmatic, Get Checked for GERD

Asthmatics who frequently awaken during sleep need to be checked for possible GERD. Asthmatics have twitchy airways. The condition is an inflammation of the bronchial tubes, and it's characterized by progressive narrowing of the tubes, accumulation of mucus, and swelling of the airways. In an asthma attack, the breathing tubes go into spasm and constrict. Asthma sufferers wheeze because of pushing air through airways that go from small to smaller; it becomes like trying to breathe through a straw. During the day, these symptoms may seem completely under control, particularly with the regular use of inhaled corticosteroids, but many patients find they return at night with a vengeance. The asthmatic is left wondering, "I did everything right, so why can't I sleep?" It could be an undiagnosed case of GERD.

280. If Asthma Symptoms Awaken You, Ask Your Partner If You Snore

Untreated snoring and sleep apnea can contribute to nocturnal symptoms of asthma. While the exact connection is not entirely clear, the vibrating soft palate may trigger airway inflammation with resultant narrowing of the bronchial tubes. Treatment of your snoring and obstructive sleep apnea may lead to better asthma control and fewer nocturnal awakenings. Additionally, untreated obstructive sleep apnea can contribute to reflux. As you try to suck in air through a collapsed, obstructed airway, you may be sucking acid into the esophagus. Treatment of obstructive sleep apnea may lead to improvement in your reflux.

281. Remember the Rule of 2s for Asthma

If you awaken more than two nights a month from your asthma, then it is not adequately controlled. Under the influence of circadian rhythms, bronchial airway narrowing increases at night. For the asthmatic who may have inflamed airways with mucus accumulation, this added narrowing can lead to nocturnal awakenings with coughing and shortness of breath. These episodes can be frightening and life threatening. If you are awakening at night because of your asthma, talk to your physician or health care provider about a "step up" in therapy. First-line therapy for persistent asthma in children and adults is inhaled corticosteroid therapy.

282. Get a Thyroid Test

Get a thyroid test if you feel tired and have gained weight with no clear explanation. A malfunctioning thyroid may lead to symptoms like feeling cold, constipation, dry skin, fatigue, and sleep apnea. About three percent of patients with obstructive sleep apnea have hypothyroidism, a condition that's easily addressed with medication.

283. Use Light Therapy for SADness That Interferes with Sleep

The kind of light therapy device that helps people with sleep phase syndromes may also alleviate the symptoms of seasonal affective disorder (SAD), which is a mood disorder associated with wintertime, and its diminished sunlight. SAD can affect sleep in the same way non-seasonal depression can disrupt it: When people feel as though they have little to live for, they can suffer nightmares, or just generally have restless sleep. Light therapy in the morning can convince the brain that it should think about summer vacation, not shoveling snow.

284. Get a Prostate Exam If You Are a Man over Fifty

Men fifty and older should get regular checkups for prostate problems to avoid waking up at night with the urge to urinate. When a man hits fifty, he becomes increasingly vulnerable to having an enlarged prostate. The prostate sits right under the bladder and surrounds the urethra, where urine exits from the bladder. An enlarged prostate squeezes around the urethra and makes it difficult for the man to empty his bladder completely, so he feels as though he has to go to the bathroom a lot, including at night. Avoid the problem by getting regular checkups.

285. See a Urologist If You Have Painful Nocturnal Erections

As we mentioned earlier, it is normal for men to have erections during REM sleep. Men commonly awaken with an erection in the morning because they have awakened out of REM sleep. Very rarely, painful erections can develop during REM sleep. This can be both physically and psychologically distressing. It is a difficult problem to treat, but if you develop it, do not be embarrassed to speak to your physician about it. He or she will probably refer you to a urologist.

286. Exercise If You Have Fibromyalgia

Fibromyalgia is a condition characterized by diffuse muscle and joint discomfort. Although not progressive or deadly, fibromyalgia syndrome (FS) plagues 10 to 11 million Americans. Multiple tender points are usually present. Sleep is often fragmented and this contributes to daytime fatigue. "Exercise" is a frightening concept for many people with FS. Exercise can reduce symptoms, increase functionality, and improve your mood, all of which lead to a better daytime and nighttime. The exercise program must reflect what you personally need and enjoy, however, not what other people in the gym are doing—no sudden moves requiring a lot of force, no bouncing, no high repetition sets. Designed by a certified personal trainer with a clinical exercise specialty, the program for an FS sufferer focuses on "health training," not "weight training" or "sports training." The key to your success is consistency, not how much you sweat or how much money you spend on a gym membership. In fact, some of the best exercises can easily be done at home. Walking, moving around in water, gentle stretching, cycling, and other non-impact or low-impact activities will help. If you have access to a pool, just make sure it's warm (84–90°F) because the FS tends to lower tolerance to cold water. Invest in at least a couple of sessions with that qualified trainer to get an initial assessment and a program that matches your abilities and goals. Ideally, you would continue to work with a pro, but since that's not an option for everyone, at least be sure to come back to the trainer periodically to make the necessary adjustments based on your progress. Medicines and cognitive behavioral therapy can also decrease symptoms of fibromyalgia.

287. Get Checked for Chronic Fatigue Syndrome

If you have no energy, you should get checked for chronic fatigue syndrome (CFS). If you have felt fatigued for no apparent reason for months, and you find that resting and sleeping do not help, then consider whether or not you have any of the other signs of chronic fatigue syndrome:

- Decreased short term memory and concentration
- Sore throat
- Tender lymph nodes in the neck or armpits
- Muscle pain
- Pain in the joints without swelling
- Headaches
- Unrefreshing sleep
- Post-exertion malaise lasting more than twenty-four hours

According to the Centers for Disease Control (CDC), if you have four or more of these symptoms for six months, then you might have CFS. It is more common in women. While the cause of CFS has not been firmly established, it may be related to an underlying chronic inflammatory process. Medicines such as selective serotonin reuptake inhibitors, or tricyclic antidepressants sometimes help, and non-steroidal anti-inflammatory drugs may relieve some of the pain. Stimulant therapy may also help. Although many CFS sufferers do not find the thought of exercise appealing, studies have indicated an exercise program can reduce symptoms, including improving the quality of sleep.

Clinical exercise specialists generally work with the CFS patient's doctor to create a program. Patients with chronic fatigue syndrome are not necessarily sleepy, by the way.

288. Try Wrist Splints to Treat Carpal Tunnel Syndrome

Carpal tunnel syndrome is a common cause of nocturnal hand and arm pain. Carpal tunnel syndrome is caused by irritation of a nerve called the median nerve where it passes through a narrow space (the carpal tunnel) at the wrist. This can produce numbness, tingling, and pain in the thumb and first two fingers, often with radiation into the arm. These symptoms are usually worse at night. Carpal tunnel syndrome is often transiently present during pregnancy; it is also seen more frequently in diabetics. If you are diagnosed with carpal tunnel syndrome by your internist or a neurologist, you can be treated in several ways. The approach to try first is to purchase wrist splints at a local drugstore. These splints are worn at night (and sometimes during the day) to maintain the wrist in a position which puts the least amount of traction on the nerve. Wearing these splints at night may be all you need to do to relieve your symptoms. If this is not successful, more aggressive treatments include steroid injection at the wrist, or hand surgery to "release" the nerve.

289. Change Position If You Wake Up with Tingling Fingers

Another nerve which can misbehave at night is the ulnar nerve. This nerve passes very close to the surface of the skin and can be pinched or compressed at the elbow. It is vulnerable to being compressed when you lie on your back with arms outstretched. If your 4th and 5th fingers tingle and "fall asleep," causing you to wake up, turning from your back to your side should alleviate the problem.

290. Sleep with Your Oxygen If You Have Chronic Obstructive Pulmonary Disease

If you have COPD, your physician may prescribe oxygen for nighttime use. While not all patients with COPD require oxygen therapy at night, some will develop significant drops in oxygenation due to changes associated with impairment in lung function in combination with the normal physiologic changes of breathing during sleep. Prolonged drops in oxygen during sleep can put a strain on the heart and can contribute to a heart attack, stroke, or fatal cardiac arrhythmias. If your physician has determined that your oxygen level does decrease during sleep, be sure to wear your oxygen every night. Discuss with your physician whether you will need to do the same when you are away from home. If necessary, delivery of oxygen can be arranged when you are away from home. This will definitely require advance planning. If your physician has determined that you do require oxygen during sleep, regular use can prolong your life.

291. Ask Your Doctor to Prescribe Humidification

If the oxygen you wear at night for COPD causes nasal drying, ask your physician to prescribe humidification. This can be provided with a specifically designed bottle of water connected to the oxygen tank in your bedroom.

292. If You Have Congestive Heart Failure, Watch for Leg Swelling

Patients with congestive heart failure (CHF) need to watch for the development of leg swelling. Leg swelling in patients with CHF is a sign of too much fluid in the body. The heart is a pump, and when the pump loses so much tone that it doesn't do its job well, the condition is called congestive heart failure. The heart struggles to get blood that contains oxygen and vital nutrients into the body, and fluid backs up into the legs and lungs. When the CHF patient goes to bed, a lot of the fluid contained in the legs can re-enter the system and cause paroxysmal nocturnal dyspnea (PND), severe shortness of breath that wakes the person up. A fit of coughing and wheezing might follow, and that makes going back to sleep a major challenge. Not infrequently, patients will sit up on the side of the bed or seek comfort sitting on a chair. The presence of swelling in the legs, or the shortness of breath as described, suggests that your physician will need to adjust your medication to improve your heart function and to decrease your body's extra fluid.

293. Avoid Fast Foods If You Have CHF

The high salt content of many fast foods will lead to fluid accumulation if you have congestive heart failure. This can contribute to sleep disruption from paroxysmal nocturnal dyspnea. Dietary indiscretion, including increased salt intake, is one of the most common causes of worsening fluid retention in congestive heart failure.

294. If You Have CHF, Take Your Medications

If you have congestive heart failure, skipping medications can contribute to deteriorating heart function and fluid accumulation. This can lead to sleep disruption and serious cardiac problems.

295. If You Have CHF, Don't Take Diuretics Before Bed

Patients with CHF and on diuretics need to insure they take diuretics in the morning and not before bedtime. A lot of patients on multiple medications try to mitigate the adverse reactions by taking the meds at night. They find that whatever nausea or dizziness may show up as a side effect doesn't seem to matter as much if they are tucked in bed. And so they line up the pills and take everything at night, including the diuretics. The diuretics will still work just fine, of course. Right in the middle of a dream about vacationing in Tahiti, you wake up with the powerful urge to take a trip to the bathroom. If your physician has prescribed a diuretic to be taken twice a day, ask if you can take the second dose in the afternoon rather than at bedtime.

296. Stack Your Pillows

The symptom of orthopnea, or inability to lie flat because of shortness of breath, can develop in patients with congestive heart failure. This is often a sign of deteriorating heart function or excessive fluid accumulation. If you develop orthopnea, while you may find relief by adding additional pillows, you should call your physician to determine whether an adjustment in your medical therapy is required. Rarely, neurologic disorders involving the diaphragm can manifest as orthopnea.

297. Evaluate Chest Pain Immediately

Any suspicion of coronary artery disease—use the sleep-related signs here as a guide—and you should get help immediately. The number one killer in the United States is myocardial infarction: heart attack. This is due to occlusion of one the tiny vessels in your heart known as the coronary arteries. Progressive obstruction occurs over many years. When narrowing becomes advanced or a piece of plaque ruptures, symptoms may include awakening with chest pain or shortness of breath. You must seek immediate medical attention if this occurs. Contributing factors to coronary artery disease include smoking, obesity, diabetes, hypertension, increased cholesterol, advancing age, and a family history.

298. If You Have Parkinson's Disease, Discuss Sleep Problems with Your Neurologist

Patients with Parkinson's disease often complain of restless sleep. They may be uncomfortable at night due to difficulty in moving in bed. They also have an increased likelihood of having periodic limb movements and REM Sleep Behavior Disorder. Their sleep at night may be compromised by excessive sleep during the daytime. Patients with Parkinson's disease may have other unrelated sleep disorders including sleep apnea. If you are a Parkinson's disease patient with sleep difficulty, contact your neurologist and be specific about what you are experiencing.

299. Seek Help If You Are Having Difficulty Caring for a Relative with Alzheimer's Disease Who Is "Sundowning"

Patients with dementia such as Alzheimer's disease may become more agitated and disoriented at night, a phenomenon called "sundowning." In severe cases, such patients can have a nearly complete reversal of the normal sleep-wake cycle. Ask the patient's physician for insights and help.

300. Try a Bilevel Pressure Unit if You Have a Nerve or Muscle Disorder Causing Weakness

Certain disorders such as ALS (amyotrophic lateral sclerosis) can cause weakness of the muscles of breathing. During sleep, with the skeletal muscle paralysis that we all experience, we rely heavily on the main breathing muscle known as the diaphragm. This muscle has two parts, one under each lung. As this muscle contracts, air flows into the lungs. If the diaphragm is weakened due to a nerve or muscle disorder, it may not be able to handle the increased load during sleep while other breathing muscles are paralyzed. Recall that during REM sleep, skeletal muscle paralysis occurs. Bilevel positive airway pressure may provide the extra support needed by the diaphragm by decreasing the effort needed to draw in air. Typically, a neurologist and pulmonologist work closely together to treat these conditions requiring bilevel pressure. (For more discussion of bilevel pressure devices, see Chapter 6: Advice for People Who Snore.)

301. Look Into Therapy If You Have PTSD

If you have served in battle, witnessed or been the victim of violent crime, or had any other kind of traumatic experience, then you might have post traumatic stress disorder (PTSD). If you have PTSD, you may have difficulty falling asleep or staying asleep. Your body has put you on alert for danger: You have an increased sense of fight or flight. Nightmares, panic attacks, flashbacks to the traumatic event and heightened sensitivity to noise can disturb your rest. In addition to telling your physician or health care provider, stay away from alcohol and drugs, unless the medication has been prescribed for you.

302. Get Help for Depression

If you have early morning awakening and lack of motivation, you may be depressed. Symptoms of depression include:

- Feelings of sadness
- Feelings of guilt
- Feelings of worthlessness
- Inability to concentrate
- Loss of ability to enjoy life
- Crying spells
- Thoughts of hurting yourself

If you are experiencing some of these symptoms, it is likely that depression is a contributing factor to your sleep disruption. A classic symptom is awakening in the middle of the night with an inability to return to sleep. Many factors can contribute to depression. Stresses such as job loss, divorce, or death of a loved one may contribute. Childhood traumas can linger and resurface from time to time. Additionally, biochemical imbalance in your brain's regulation of the neurotransmitter, serotonin, may be playing a role. Professional counseling and antidepressant medication may be extremely helpful. Seek out medical care immediately if you have thoughts about hurting yourself.

303. Get Checked for an Ulcer

If abdominal pain wakes you up at night, you may have an ulcer. Corrosive acids in the stomach are secreted to break down food that we ingest. Sometimes these acids can cause an erosion of the stomach lining or ulcer, or even a hole in the stomach or part of the small intestine known as the duodenum. When acid contacts the erosion, it can be very painful. Patients with ulcers often have an increased production of acid while sleeping. This may lead to nocturnal awakening with abdominal pain. Antacids, ranitidine, and proton pump inhibitors may provide relief. However, in severe cases, profuse bleeding or life-threatening perforation of the stomach or duodenum may occur. Therefore, don't just treat this condition with over-the-counter medicines, see your physician or health care provider before a serious problem develops.

304. You May Need a Ventilator If You Have a Spinal Cord Injury

If you have an injury high in your spinal cord, you may require a ventilator during sleep. The spinal cord delivers important nerve impulses from your brain to your muscles. The level of spinal cord injury determines which muscles are impaired.

Higher injuries in the cervical spine can interfere with nerve impulses to the diaphragm. If this occurs, the diaphragm is unable to handle the work of breathing during sleep. In this situation, a tracheostomy is performed. A ventilator delivering oxygen and removing carbon dioxide is attached to the opening of the tracheostomy tube. In some patients, the ventilator may not be necessary during the day as other intact muscles handle the workload of breathing. Ventilators in the home require a dedicated family, nursing staff, and pulmonary physician.

305. If You Had Polio, Get Evaluated for Sleep-Related Breathing Problems

If you had polio decades ago, but now awaken unrefreshed, or with a headache, get evaluated for a sleep-related breathing problem. With the development of the polio vaccine in 1952, the incidence of this dreaded disease decreased significantly. However, if you suffered from polio prior to the vaccine being available, you could develop post-polio syndrome decades later. Symptoms may include awakening in the morning with a headache, daytime fatigue, muscle weakness, and difficulty breathing with activity. During sleep, your muscles may not be strong enough to sustain adequate breathing. See your physician or health care provider to discuss getting a sleep study. You may benefit from the breathing support provided by a bilevel pressure device while you sleep.

306. Get Checked for Hyperthyroidism

Always feeling warm and nervous, losing your hair, and can't sleep? Ask your physician or health care provider to check for hyperthyroidism. A simple blood test can determine if your thyroid gland (responsible for your body's metabolism) is overactive and secreting too much thyroid hormone. This stimulating hormone can contribute to difficulty initiating and maintaining sleep. Treatment often involves an endocrinologist who specializes in management of gland disorders. Medications are often highly effective in treating this condition.

307. Find Out the Source of Nocturnal Choking

If you awaken in the middle of the night choking, you may have sleep apnea. But you should also consider other possible causes including:

- **Laryngospasm.** When the vocal cords are stimulated with acid from reflux, they go into spasm and block off your airway. This frightening symptom can last for seconds to minutes, but usually resolves while you sit terrified on the edge of your bed. Reflux is discussed further in the tips above.
- **Paroxysmal Nocturnal Dyspnea.** See tips relating to congestive heart failure.
- **Panic attacks.** If you are under a lot of stress or suffer from generalized anxiety, you may be awakening with a smothering feeling related to acute anxiety during sleep. Once your physician or health care provider has excluded a more serious medical condition, focusing on your underlying stresses is essential.

9

Advice for People on
Prescription Medications

308. Adjust Your Dosage to Minimize Impact on Sleep

309. Ask Your Physician about a Non-Sedating Antihistamine

310. Take Your Diuretics Earlier in the Day

311. If You Are on Diuretics and Have Leg Cramps, Get Your Electrolytes Checked

312. Be Aware of the Effects of Antidepressants on Sleep

313. If You Have Chronic Insomnia, Check Your Depression Medication

314. Check Your Asthma Medication If You Have Trouble Sleeping

315. Be Careful Using Benzodiazepines

316. Try a Different Medication If Your Beta Blocker Makes You Sleepy or Causes Insomnia

317. Be Careful with Cold Medication

318. Ask for a Sleeping Pill During a Difficult Time

319. If Arthritis Keeps You Up, Ask for an Anti-Inflammatory Medication

Factors discussed here are medications that affect sleep by cutting it short, altering the experience of sleep, prolonging it beyond what you consider desirable, or causing sleep unexpectedly. Medication should help you regain full functioning, not rob you of it. For many conditions, effective medications with different mechanisms of action and different side effect profiles are now available. Work with your physician or health care provider to find the right one for you.

308. Adjust Your Dosage to Minimize Impact on Sleep

Adjust when you take medications as well as the dosage to minimize impact on sleep. Along with advancing age often comes a plethora of medical conditions such as congestive heart failure, arthritis, diabetes, and reflux that may have manifestations at night that disrupt sleep. To make matters worse, the medications for these conditions can also disrupt sleep. Be sure to check with your physician before making any changes in your medical regimen.

309. Ask Your Physician about a Non-Sedating Antihistamine

Medicines that make you drowsy during the day may contribute to napping, which can disrupt your nighttime sleep. Additionally, daytime sleepiness caused by these medications may have an adverse impact on coordination, work performance, and safe driving. Allergy sufferers know that the itchy watery eyes, stuffy running nose, and hacking cough can be quite uncomfortable and lead to sleep disruption. Many new medications have been developed to alleviate these symptoms, but before taking pills or using nasal sprays, make sure that identification and avoidance of offending allergens has been considered. If symptoms persist despite these measures, non-sedating anti-inflammatory nasal sprays such as nasal steroids and eye drops such as olopatadine hydrochloride may alleviate all of your symptoms. If symptoms persist, try a non-sedating antihistamine. Many of these can be purchased over the counter. However, even though they are touted as being non-sedating, some may cause sleepiness.

310. Take Your Diuretics Earlier in the Day

Move the timing of your diuretics earlier in the day if possible. Talk with your doctor about taking diuretics earlier in the day so you can get longer periods of restful sleep. You want to avoid getting up in the middle of the night, or several times a night, in response to the diuretics.

311. If You Are on Diuretics and Have Leg Cramps, Get Your Electrolytes Checked

If you are on a diuretic, this can lead to depletion of electrolytes such as potassium and magnesium. This then can contribute to leg cramps. Your physician may want to check a blood test for your electrolytes.

312. Be Aware of the Effects of Antidepressants on Sleep

Antidepressants can affect your sleep in several ways. Some are alerting and others are sedating (see below). Most antidepressants suppress REM sleep. The reduction in REM sleep typically does not produce any functional deficits, but people on antidepressants might find that they do not recall many dreams. A reduction in REM sleep should not make you feel more tired the following day. Many antidepressants can aggravate symptoms of restless legs syndrome.

313. If You Have Chronic Insomnia, Check Your Depression Medication

You may need to revisit your depression medication if you have chronic insomnia. In the management of depression, selective serotonin reuptake inhibitors (or SSRIs) and cognitive behavioral therapy (CBT) have revolutionized medical therapy. Unfortunately, some SSRIs can cause insomnia and others can produce excessive sleepiness. If insomnia or sedation develops when you go on an SSRI, your physician may want to consider another medication. It is always important to discuss any side effects you may encounter with your medical therapy with your physician or health care provider.

314. Check Your Asthma Medication If You Have Trouble Sleeping

Many of the medicines we use to treat the bronchoconstriction of asthma have a stimulating effect. Xanthine derivatives, while still used for some patients, have been largely replaced by newer, less stimulating medications. However, even newer beta agonist containing treatments can be stimulating and lead to difficulty initiating and maintaining sleep. If you are on asthma therapy and have trouble sleeping, ask your physician or health care provider if any of your medications may be contributing.

315. Be Careful Using Benzodiazepines

You should exercise caution with the use of benzodiazepines if you have COPD. Some patients with chronic obstructive pulmonary disease have elevations in their carbon dioxide level, a byproduct of cellular metabolism. The use of benzodiazepines for sleep or anxiety could contribute to dangerous elevations of carbon dioxide. This can result in sleepiness and even coma. If you have COPD and your physician or health care provider has prescribed a benzodiazepine, immediately report any increase in sleepiness.

316. Try a Different Medication If Your Beta Blocker Makes You Sleepy or Causes Insomnia

If a beta blocker prescribed to you for high blood pressure makes you sleepy, or alternatively seems to produce insomnia, ask your physician to try a different medication. Hypertension has a well-deserved reputation as the silent killer. It is a major contributing factor in the development of a heart attack, stroke, and end-stage renal disease requiring dialysis. Many effective medications have been developed to treat your high blood pressure, so work with your doctor to find a medical regimen that works for you without causing intolerable side effects. Note that weight loss, alcohol avoidance, exercise, salt restriction, and treatment of obstructive sleep apnea are other measures that can improve your hypertension. The great benefit is that these measures may decrease the need for medication therapy. You should discuss these alternative interventions with your physician or health care provider.

317. Be Careful with Cold Medication

"Common cold" medicines vary; choose carefully in treating your upper respiratory tract infection. Be careful with over-the-counter preparations when you have the common cold. Everyone has experienced the annoying symptoms of an upper respiratory tract infection. Nasal stuffiness, drippy running nose, sore throat, and aches are often experienced when you are sick with a "cold." In the absence of high fever, dark yellow phlegm production, or an underlying serious medical condition, you most likely are suffering from a self-limited viral illness that will not benefit from antibiotic therapy. Associated symptoms of your cold may keep you up at night. Be sure to read the label of your over-the-counter medication. Some of these medicines cause daytime sleepiness. Some of these medicines can cause stimulation that leads to sleep disruption. Consider short-term use of acetaminophen for low-grade fevers, aches and discomfort. A cough syrup containing dextromethorphan can be quite helpful. If your cough persists and disrupts sleep despite this, a narcotic prescribed by your physician or health care provider for temporary bedtime use can be extremely helpful. If you do take a narcotic at bedtime, be careful with driving the next day. Ultimately, the best treatment for your upper respiratory tract infection is "a tincture of time."

318. Ask for a Sleeping Pill During a Difficult Time

If you've been diagnosed with a life-threatening disease, ask for a sleeping pill to help you get through the trauma of the diagnosis. Being diagnosed with a serious illness can have a profound and traumatic impact on your entire life, including your sleep. If you are returning to your physician or health care provider for test results that may include the possibility of an upsetting diagnosis, come prepared for the office visit:

- Bring a family member or close relative who can serve as a secretary to record what you are told.

- Bring a list of questions you undoubtedly have, but will likely forget to ask after hearing the diagnosis.
- Ask for a sleeping pill. You may have trouble sleeping once you hear the new diagnosis. Even if you don't have trouble sleeping, you will be comforted knowing that you have a pill to help you sleep if you need it. This in itself may improve your sleep. You don't want this acute trauma to lead to insomnia that could persist for years after your illness has been cured.

319. If Arthritis Keeps You Up, Ask for an Anti-Inflammatory Medication

The pain and inflammation of arthritis can lead to disabling immobility. It can also lead to significant sleep disruption as you try to find a comfortable position. With new advances in medical therapy, you need not suffer. Your physician or health care provider will want to determine what type of arthritis you have, and then tailor a treatment regimen with medications and exercise specifically for you. Sometimes a steroid injection can provide considerable relief for a problematic, painful area.

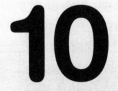

10

Advice on
Alternative Therapies

320. Aim for Realignment with a Chiropractic Adjustment

321. Find a Practitioner of TCM to Explore Your Insomnia

322. Try Acupuncture, but Be Patient

323. Ask Your Acupuncturist about Electro-Acupuncture

324. Try Acupressure

325. Make Sure Your Herbal Tea Is Caffeine-Free

326. Choose Calcium in Your Pre-Bed Snack

327. Try Oyster Shells

328. Magnesium May Help You Relax

329. Try Melatonin

330. Research the Benefits of Different Types of Tea

331. Be Cautious If You Try Valerian

332. Be Careful with Siberian Ginseng

333. Avoid Gelsemium

334. Try Coffea, Not Coffee

335. Reach for a Little Bowl of Berries

336. Get to the Points with Massage Therapy

337. Massage Yourself

355. Spend Time with People You Enjoy

356. Cuddle a Body Pillow to Stop Sleeping on Your Stomach

357. Try Biofeedback Exercises

358. Calm Down with Lavender

359. Try Other Flower Essences, Too

360. Discover What Type of Aromatherapy Works Best for You

361. If You Like Sleeping on Your Back, Try a Knee Wedge

362. And Speaking of Your Back, Enjoy a Back Scratch

363. Use a Contoured Knee Pillow to Make Sleeping on Your Side More Comfortable

364. Seek Help from a Certified Hypnotherapist for Your Occasional Insomnia

365. Seek Additional Sources of Information

Some of the tips in this chapter reflect good advice from exercise specialists, and some come from physical therapists, so in that sense, it isn't all what you might deem "alternative." Nevertheless, these are not necessarily tips you would get from physicians, so we have placed them in this chapter.

We also want to make it clear that the advice in this chapter on topics related to Traditional Chinese Medicine and chiropractic, for example, comes from interviews with people who have knowledge of it, and not from physicians associated with a sleep center. At the outset, though, we did notice how much of the foundation advice on sleep hygiene is compatible with a Western medicine approach. We all agree on the need to prepare for sleep with quiet time, reserving the bed for sleeping and sex only, soothing yourself with a cup of herbal tea, and many other tips.

Also, we don't want to diminish the value of alternative therapies, so if you want more in-depth insights, then go directly to the people who have it at organizations such as the American Chiropractic Association, The American Association of Acupuncture Oriental Medicine, American Herbal Products Association, American Botanical Council, and American Massage Therapy Association, as well as to your local certified physical therapists, massage therapists, and personal trainers—and this is, by no means, an exhaustive list of sources and personal resources.

320. Aim for Realignment with a Chiropractic Adjustment

A study published in the Journal of Manipulative and Physiological Therapeutics (Volume 28, Issue 3, Pages 179–186, March 2005, J. Jamison) attempted to answer the question "Insomnia: Does Chiropractic Help?" Interestingly, the fifteen chiropractors who participated in the study were a lot more hesitant than the patients in suggesting there were benefits. One-third of the 154 patients in the study reported that they had immediate benefit from their series of adjustments.

321. Find a Practitioner of TCM to Explore Your Insomnia

Practitioners of Traditional Chinese Medicine (TCM) consider insomnia a flag signaling another underlying problem—not unlike practitioners of Western medicine, as you can see from the tips related to conditions like allergies, nasal obstruction, and so on. In trying to find patterns that may underlie your sleeping problems, a TCM practitioner would consider problems such as parasites, anemia, blood sugar problems, constipation, liver problems, heart problems, and stress. This is similar to the approach taken by practitioners of Western medicine in looking for underlying causes of sleep disturbances. For example, the advice on iron deficiency given in the tips on Restless Legs Syndrome and pregnancy in earlier chapters is consistent in principle with what you would get from a practitioner of alternative medicine.

322. Try Acupuncture, but Be Patient

Acupuncture involves placing needles at specific locations on the body to treat problems and promote health. It can be used to treat insomnia, with the practitioner placing the needles with the aim of soothing the nervous system. But the balancing and calming effects apparently do take multiple sessions, so in fairness to your practitioner, you should walk in expecting to schedule repeat visits to address your sleep issues.

323. Ask Your Acupuncturist about Electro-Acupuncture

Ask your acupuncturist about electro-acupuncture to reduce the time commitment. In electro-acupuncture therapy, the practitioner attaches electrodes to the needles that are inserted under your skin. This provides continuous movement of the needle in the area, thereby giving the practitioner's hand a break. The technique should reduce the amount of time it takes to complete a treatment.

324. Try Acupressure

According to acupressure experts, if you want quick relief, try putting pressure at two points on your arm—one at your wrist just below your little finger, and one right about the center of your lower arm area (near the wrist) between the major bones. You approach them from the inner wrist, so this is something you could do easily while lying in bed.

325. Make Sure Your Herbal Tea Is Caffeine-Free

Make sure to check the labels to be sure that your herbal tea is caffeine free. With the world full of great tea options, it's easy to make assumptions that "herbal" means "caffeine free," but that's not necessarily so.

326. Choose Calcium in Your Pre-Bed Snack

If you don't like warm milk, try tofu. Other than the warmth of the milk, another reason why it may serve as a good nightcap is the calcium content, which some practitioners believe may work as a natural sedative. There are good dairy and non-dairy sources of calcium, so maybe you would rather have a cup of yogurt or a bowl of peas as your light pre-bed snack.

327. Try Oyster Shells

Oyster shell, which is readily available in vitamin stores in both tablet and liquid delivery systems, also contains calcium and is used to help reduce sleep problems. Have a little food with it, though, and if you are on any prescription medications, be sure to tell your doctor you want to add this to your daily diet. Same guidance applies to all supplements listed here.

328. Magnesium May Help You Relax

One manifestation of a magnesium deficiency is a kind of restlessness that could delay getting to sleep. Try a supplement, but you may want to take this with a light snack to avoid stomach upset, as manufacturers tend to recommend. If you have kidney disease, taking this supplemental mineral could be dangerous and must be monitored carefully by your physician or health care provider.

329. Try Melatonin

You can try melatonin, but with caution. Melatonin has the ability to disturb your circadian rhythm, cause a kind of hangover, and increase symptoms of depression, among other things. Start with a low dosage—about 1.5 mg—and then if you conclude that you want a greater effect, increase the dosage conservatively. Do not exceed 6 mg a day, though, and do not take it if you are pregnant or under the care of a doctor for any serious medical condition.

330. Research the Benefits of Different Types of Tea

Tea may offer more benefits than warmth. Chamomile and lemon verbena tea may have value in helping you rest because of the relaxing effect of the herbs in addition to the warmth of the tea.

331. Be Cautious If You Try Valerian

Valerian may help ease you into sleep, or keep you awake. Valerian can be ingested in different ways, such as extracts, tablets, and capsules. One popular option is to use it in tea. Because valerian has developed a reputation for being effective in treating insomnia—a fact that the National Institutes of Health has not conclusively confirmed with available studies, but lukewarmly suggests may be true in some cases—the nick-name for valerian is "herbal Valium." Note, however, that valerian and Valium, which is a synthetic sedative, have no relationship at all. Also, it is a well-documented fact that valerian does not have a calming effect on everyone. Some people find it stimulating. So go easy in trying it: Take a dosage less than the one recommended on the bottle and, if it makes you a little tired, then take the full dosage at bedtime.

332. Be Careful with Siberian Ginseng

Stay away from Siberian Ginseng to reduce signs of stress if you have high blood pressure. Ginseng is one of the many confusing herbal supplements on the market because it has been touted as a cure for so many problems. To complicate matters, there are different types of ginseng and the quality of products on the market range from poor to excellent. (Check with sources like the American Botanical Council for information on standards.) Siberian Ginseng has gained some popularity with people undergoing radiation treatment for cancer and people suffering from fibromyalgia and chronic fatigue syndrome. In theory, if you can beat back the ill effects of the treatment or the condition by using it, then you will have more refreshing sleep. Unfortunately, this is not a product that people with high blood pressure should even consider taking as it raises blood pressure. If you are being treated for high blood pressure, do not use it. Also, this is not something you would take right before bedtime.

333. Avoid Gelsemium

Typical uses of this substance have been for dull headaches and for temporary insomnia related to issues that give you dull headaches like "Will I do well on that job interview in the morning?" It has long been considered unsafe for use by pregnant women, but recently there is widespread skepticism about whether it should be used by anyone. The remedy is named after the toxic plant that is the main active ingredient.

334. Try Coffea, Not Coffee

Coffea, not coffee, could help. The homeopathic remedy coffea cruda is used by some practitioners of natural medicine to treat insomnia. Ironically, the remedy actually is coffee-based, but it's unroasted coffee.

335. Reach for a Little Bowl of Berries

Or put them on the cereal you're having as a late snack. Berries turn to sugar a lot more slowly than most other fruits, so they won't give you a big rush of energy and you'll get the benefit of a comfort food with good vitamins.

336. Get to the Points with Massage Therapy

Massage therapists trying to help you address your insomnia will likely go to five different points on your body to help relieve conditions that may be disrupting your sleep. They will probably massage the back of the neck, an area midway between your navel and your chest, close to the pubic area, mid back, and lower back.

337. Massage Yourself

Human beings have certain body language in common regardless of ethnic origin or gender. Body movements called adaptors are gestures that relieve stress and comfort the body. Generally, they are rubbing movements, such as a baseball player rubbing his legs before batting, or an executive rubbing her neck before giving a presentation to the board of directors. Knowing that these movements relieve stress, you can consciously do them to help you relax before bedtime. Applying body lotion and using a shower sponge are two ways to "adapt" before you head for bed.

338. Mirror Your Cat and Dog

Some people find gentle stretching to be helpful before bed. The Cat/Dog Stretch both stretches and strengthens your abdominal muscles and spine to create a relaxed feeling. Kneel on the carpet by your bed and put your hands flat in front of you. Round your back and let your head hang down. Stretch as you look toward your navel; that's the cat. Look up toward the ceiling and arch your back as you lift your head upward; that's the dog. Repeat this ten times. Inhale as you become your dog. Exhale as you become your cat.

339. Get a Leg Up on Sleep

Actually get two legs up to relieve legs and feet. Lie on the carpet next to your bed and let your legs rest straight up at the 90-degree angle to your body. Straighten the knees as much as possible, while keeping your arms relaxed at your sides. Breathe easily. Doing straight leg stretches with easy breathing like this before bedtime will help you avoid episodic nocturnal cramps as well as calm your mind and your body.

340. Bend Like Gumby

Remember that dark green humanoid TV character named Gumby that came into your home as a bendable toy? Well now he's going to teach you something.

Interlock your fingers behind your back and bend forward. Let your head fall into a relaxed position toward your knees. You can slightly bend your knees if keeping the legs straight puts too much strain on the back of your legs. Stretch your arms toward the ceiling and hold that for about 20 seconds, then stand up. It's a great chest stretch that should make you feel as though you're breathing a little easier.

341. Stretch Like a Pigeon

You can store a great deal of tension in the area around your hips because of sitting at a desk, and generally doing things that never stretch your hip area. Your sleeping may be much more comfortable if you relieve stress in that area. Get on the floor and bend your right leg inward, so you can put your left breast (or left side of your chest) on, or close to, your right knee. Collapse so that your arms are outstretched above your head, your head droops down and you feel as though your back is fully stretched. Move that right foot to increase the comfort level. If you are not dealing with significant weight or flexibility issues, you should be able to get into a position that feels completely relaxing. Repeat that with the opposite leg/chest combination. Hold each one for twenty seconds, or even longer if you feel truly comfortable in the position. This is called a "sleeping pigeon" position.

342. Get Into Your Sleep Position

Some people find comfort in assuming a fetal position for sleeping, whereas others like to sprawl on their back. It won't be the same every time, but there may be one position more than others that you associate with sleep. Get into it and enjoy the sensation of relaxing into a restful sleep. "Assuming the position" could be nothing more than a psychological trigger for you that it's time to sleep, but if it works for you, then rely on it.

343. Have Sex

The intense pleasure of sexual activity can lead to a state of deep relaxation highly conducive to sleep onset. For some people, though, sex leads to a persistent state of arousal that can interfere with sleep onset. The key is communication with your partner. Coordinate the timing of sexual activity so that it is both enjoyable and conducive to good sleep. And don't have sex with someone who causes anxiety for you. At least, not right before you want to sleep.

344. Pick Your PJs Well — or Not

While many of us enjoy the feeling of a soft fabric at night in the form of pajamas or a nightgown, a lot of people prefer to be naked. Their favorite soft fabric is a sheet. The key word in both scenarios is "soft"—meaning non-irritating—and it can be achieved with a synthetic, as well as a natural fabric. When you buy the PJs or sheet, wash them before use and dry them without any added smells, like the ones you get from some dryer sheets, unless you associate that particular smell with sleep.

345. Reduce Your Anxiety Through Conversation and Control

You might lie in bed and worry about money, relationships, illness, work, and whether or not your car will make it through another winter. Even happy things like a wedding or new job can cause anxiety. You can take action by talking with people you trust, including health care professionals, but you can also mitigate the anxiety by taking positive action related to the anxiety-producing issues. Remember: Worry alone does nothing but make you feel bad. Cut up a high interest credit card. Make an appointment with someone at your new job who can mentor you. Take your car to a mechanic for a checkup. Get yourself unstuck from the anxiety by looking forward to things you can do to improve the situation—and then do them.

346. Process Your Thoughts about Your Dreams When You Wake Up

You can get up with a burst of energy and jump into your running shoes or get up with a sigh and drag yourself to the shower, but you don't have to do either one the second you wake up. Take a moment and contemplate what you just saw in dreamland. You may learn something about why you feel you had a good night's sleep, or a bad one.

347. Dream with Understanding

There are a number of theories about the function and meaning of dreams. Ultimately the significance of dreams remains a scientific mystery. Certain images tend to recur in dreams and in a collective sort of way, may have the same meanings. But each dreamer has dreams that are meant only for that person and must be interpreted in that light. Carolyn Wills, a former pastor and an instructor in lucid dreaming that we talked with, said this: "If you dream about a member of the clergy, it will have one meaning, but for me, it is a matter of work. If I dream about fields of corn and wheat, the significance will vary between you and me if you happen to be a farmer."

348. Dream with Control

There is a school of thought that believes in lucid dreaming as a therapeutic modality. In a lucid dream, you know you're dreaming. You can affect what happens in the dream to some extent. This is a practice that has helped people with post-traumatic stress disorder (PTSD), as well as people who have more garden-variety anxieties. If you have troubling dreams, try to take control. Go to sleep with the thought in your head that certain moments—and if you suffer from PTSD, it would be moments that you have mentally seen over and over again—can be interrupted and changed as you see them in your dreams. You will be thinking, "This is a dream. I can make it different."

349. Dream with Direction

Many people have also reported the ability to dream something that they want to dream, so they set out on their sleep path with that in mind. One way this might happen is to resume sleep after a short interruption with the thought in mind, "I'd like to go back to where I was in that dream…" and then they fall asleep and resume the dream. Another possibility is to be so well-practiced in directed dreaming that you see what you want to see, in a sense. The best way to describe it may be that you experience a short movie of your own design—with some surprises.

350. Make the Most of Your Dreaming

Develop habits to make the most of your dreaming. These steps come from Carolyn Wills, who has taught directed dreaming and abided by these principles for decades:

1. Write down your dreams. Keep a notebook at your bedside. Scribble in the dark—you'll figure it out later.
2. Name the dream. What is the central theme? What emotions did you feel as you recorded it? Take your dreams seriously.
3. Pay attention to repetitions. When a dream repeats itself, or an event within a dream repeats itself, it is important.

351. Laugh

The benefits of laughter have been known for centuries. In our day-to-day stressful lives, laughter can clearly prove beneficial and help decrease the stresses that contribute to sleep disruption. Rent a funny movie, watch a funny show, read a funny book.

352. Think, and Write, Positively

Take the time every day to generate a list of the things for which you are grateful. A greater appreciation of all the positive things in your life may contribute to decreased stress, increased happiness, and better sleep. We often take for granted the many beautiful things in our lives while focusing on the material possessions we wish for.

353. Volunteer If You Are Now Retired

Many retirees find themselves suddenly with too much free time and inactivity. This can lead to increased napping, increased eating, and worsening of sleep. In retirement, have a plan to keep active. Consider volunteering—and that does not have to be a formal commitment to an organization. As long as you have a regular connection to the activity, it can be anything you enjoy.

354. Get Your B12 Vitamins

Especially if you're 65 or older, make sure you get your B12. All of the B vitamins are important, but a lack of B12 particularly is associated with depression, bad temper, and apathy, and in medical terms, psychiatric and cognitive disturbances as well as damage to the spinal cord. The United States Department of Agriculture reports that studies show that 9 percent of the population shows definite signs of deficiency, and another 16 percent are borderline. The problem is not just a nutritional one, since the ability to absorb the vitamin B12 in food diminishes with age. Eating cereals fortified with B vitamins is one way to get more B12 in the system, but this may be more than an eating problem if you're over sixty-five. Increasing dietary intake will not solve the problem if you cannot absorb B12 in your digestive tract. If you have symptoms of B12 deficiency, a simple blood test will determine if your B12 level is low. If you are B12-deficient and cannot absorb oral replacement, you will have to get the amount you need by injection.

355. Spend Time with People You Enjoy

The value of strong friendships cannot be overestimated in terms of helping you sleep well. Friendships engender a feeling of well-being and connection, which are vital human needs. Seek out those with whom you can share your fears and concerns. Surround yourself with people who have a positive outlook on life. It's contagious.

356. Cuddle a Body Pillow to Stop Sleeping on Your Stomach

Many of us assume the posture we did as babies and sleep on the stomach. (We now know that babies should not be placed with the belly down due to the increased risk of sudden infant death syndrome.) For some adults, sleeping on the belly can cause or contribute to back discomfort. We roll out of bed and can almost hear our vertebrae trying to straighten out after a few hours of lying face down. Invest in a long body pillow and clutch it to your front. It will simulate sleeping on your stomach without the backache in the morning.

357. Try Biofeedback Exercises

Biofeedback exercises can help you slow down. The combination of rhythmic breathing, a comfortable posture, and a mentally boring game can work together to draw you toward sleep. Pick a topic about which you know more than you wish you did: pop culture, constellations, heads of state—let your mind create lists until you fall asleep. Do this repeatedly, so that you know when you start the process that sleep will soon overtake you. You don't want to remember everyone who has won a Grammy in the past five years—you want the comfort of knowing you will fall asleep in the process of trying to remember.

358. Calm Down with Lavender

The scent of lavender provides a sense of calm, so herbalists have long recommended it as a treatment for stress. A few drops of oil in your bath might make that evening ritual even more conducive to sleep. Some people like to place a lavender tree near the bed.

359. Try Other Flower Essences, Too

Essences other than lavender can also provide calming effects; some theorize that the flower fragrances have a slight effect on brain chemistry. Your natural food store should have a good selection. The usual technique for using them is either to place a drop or two under the tongue, or add them to a beverage.

360. Discover What Type of Aromatherapy Works Best for You

There are bath oils, creams, mists, candles, incense, potpourri, and many other delivery systems of scent that you can use on your body or near your body to engender relaxation. Lavender is commonly associated with rest, but so are rose and honeysuckle, for example.

361. If You Like Sleeping On Your Back, Try A Knee Wedge

It is common during a chiropractic or massage session to have the practitioner place a pillow or foam wedge underneath your knees when you are on your back. The elevation allows your back to lie flat against the table—and it's a very relaxing sensation. Try placing a wedge, or just a folded pillow, under your knees if your preferred sleeping position is on your back.

362. And Speaking of Your Back, Enjoy a Back Scratch

A truly pleasurable and relaxing sensation is a gentle back scratch. Ask your partner to give you a light scratch as you lie down to sleep—but keep in mind that this is one of those things in which you should take turns!

363. Use a Contoured Knee Pillow to Make Sleeping on Your Side More Comfortable

People with arthritis, spinal cord injuries, and many other physical problems use this pillow that is specially shaped to fit between the knees to allow them to sleep on their side. But you don't have to have a problem to find comfort in using a knee pillow.

364. Seek Help from a Certified Hypnotherapist for Your Occasional Insomnia

If you don't have a sleep disorder such as sleep apnea or another physiological problem causing sleep disruption, you may want to consult a certified hypnotherapist. Through the National Board for Certified Clinical Hypnotherapists, you might find someone who could help you work through some of the tension that keeps you awake night after night.

365. Seek Additional Sources of Information

Information about sleep and sleep disorders is growing rapidly. We hope that this book has provided a starting point for individuals who are interested in achieving healthy sleep. We encourage you to learn more about sleep in general or about specific sleep disorders using these resources:

American Academy of Sleep Medicine: *www.aasmnet.org*
National Sleep Foundation: *www.sleepfoundation.org*
National Heart, Lung and Blood Institute: *www.nhlbi.nih.gov/health/public/sleep*

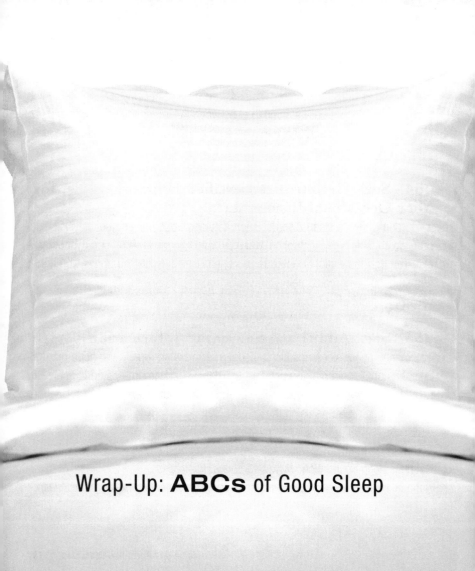

Wrap-Up: **ABCs** of Good Sleep

Airway. Treating the airway obstruction of obstructive sleep apnea will help you sleep better and feel more refreshed.

Bed. Reserve it for sleeping and sex only.

Comfort. Make it the hallmark of your sleeping arrangements.

Dreams. Enjoy them; learn to direct them.

Exercise. Aerobic activities help keep your body in balance and lead to a "good tired."

Food. Allow several hours to digest a meal before bedtime.

Gratitude. Give it to yourself and others around you to enhance your sense of peace.

Habits. Stick with your good ones, like a cup of herbal tea, at home and on the road.

Insomnia. It will happen; maintain good sleep hygiene no matter what the cause.

Joy. Do things that make you laugh, bring you comfort, and remind you of good in life.

Kids. Support their health and growth with a sleep routine.

Light. It plays a key role in circadian rhythm; keep that in mind when it's time to sleep.

Mattress. Invest in a good one, and that does not necessarily mean the most expensive one.

Naps. Take an afternoon nap if you feel the urge and have the opportunity.

Obesity. It is a major contributing factor to obstructive sleep apnea. If you are overweight, make weight loss a priority.

Positive thinking. Allow rest and dreams to come more easily by focusing on the good.

Quiet. Stay away from auditory stimuli at bedtime.

Relaxation. Wind down before you head for the bed; do something calming.

Schedules. To the extent you can, keep your bedtime regular, even if you work nights.

Therapy. Some issues will not go away without medical treatment; if you need it, get it.

Urination. It's a good thing, but if it interrupts your sleep every night, see your doctor.

Victory. You can support health and sleep by adhering to the advice in this book.

Weight. Sleep deprivation can lead to weight gain, so make good sleep part of your diet.

eXamine your sleeping environment and eliminate light and noise.

Yes. Say it when you go to bed. Accept the invitation to sleep.

Zzzzz. Sleep well.

Appendix

A

When to **Seek Help** from a **Physician**

Take the two tests below to determine if you should be evaluated for a sleep disorder.

Test #1. The Epworth Sleepiness Scale

Take this test by choosing the number that most accurately describes your likelihood to fall asleep during each situation listed, then add up your total:

0 = No chance of dozing
1 = Slight chance of dozing
2 = Moderate chance of dozing
3 = High chance of dozing

Sitting and reading
0   1   2   3

Watching TV
0   1   2   3

Sitting inactive in a public place (e.g. a theatre or meeting)
0   1   2   3

As a passenger in a car for an hour without a break
0   1   2   3

Lying down to rest in the afternoon when circumstances permit

0   1   2   3

Sitting and talking to someone

0   1   2   3

Sitting quietly after a lunch without alcohol

0   1   2   3

In a car, while stopped for a few minutes in traffic

0   1   2   3

Your Epworth total: _____

WHAT IT MEANS:

If your score is greater than 10, you are abnormally sleepy. You may place yourself or others at risk by driving or using dangerous machinery. Avoid such activities until you have seen your doctor to find out what's causing your problem.

Ask your bed partner to fill out the Epworth Sleepiness Scale with you in mind. If the score as tallied by your partner is elevated, then you may not be aware of how sleepy you are.

© M.W. Johns 1990–97

Test #2:

Answer yes or no to the following ten questions:

1. I frequently have trouble falling asleep or staying asleep. **Y** **N**
2. Despite seven to nine hours of continuous sleep, I often feel unrefreshed, sleepy, or tired during the day. **Y** **N**
3. I have been told that I kick or thrash while sleeping. **Y** **N**
4. I have an irresistible urge to rub or move my legs at night. **Y** **N**
5. I awaken from sleep with a burning sensation in my chest or throat. **Y** **N**
6. I awaken from sleep with pain or discomfort in my chest. **Y** **N**
7. I awaken from sleep with difficulty breathing. **Y** **N**
8. I have been told that I have loud disruptive snoring. **Y** **N**
9. I awaken from sleep gasping or choking. **Y** **N**
10. I have been told that I stop breathing during my sleep. **Y** **N**

If you answered Yes to any of these questions, seek help. You can begin this medical evaluation by speaking to your primary care provider, or by seeking help at an accredited Sleep Center. A list of these centers by geographical location is available at the website of the American Academy of Sleep Medicine (*www.aasmnet.org*).

Appendix

B

Insomnia Medications Table

The following table lists drugs commonly prescribed as sleep aids. You will see that many of them look familiar for two reasons: Some of them receive a lot of print and television ad space, and some of them are used primarily for other purposes, like coping with allergies and colds. These latter drugs make you drowsy, but are not approved for treating insomnia. Any drug prescribed as a hypnotic medication can produce excess sedation, and should be used with caution, particularly by elderly people. Side effects, doses, and potential drug interactions should be reviewed before any of these drugs is used.

MEDICATION	GENERIC	TYPICAL DOSE RANGE	HALF LIFE

Benzodiazepine-like hypnotics

MEDICATION	GENERIC	TYPICAL DOSE RANGE	HALF LIFE
Ambien	zolpidem	5–10 mg	2–4 hours
Sonata	zaleplon	5–10 mg	1 hour
Lunesta	eszoplicone	1–3 mg	5–7 hours

Benzodiazepines

MEDICATION	GENERIC	TYPICAL DOSE RANGE	HALF LIFE
Restoril	temazepam	15–45 mg	8–20 hours
Klonopin	clonazepam	0.5–2 mg	18–50 hours
Pro-Som	estazolam	1–2 mg	10–24 hours
Doral	quazepam	7.5–15 mg	40–70 hours
Halcion	triazolam	0.125–0.25 mg	2–4 hours
Dalmane	flurazepam	15–30 mg	50–100 hours
Valium	diazepam	5–10 mg	20–50 hours

Antidepressants

MEDICATION	GENERIC	TYPICAL DOSE RANGE	HALF LIFE
Desyrel	trazodone	50–150 mg	3–6 hours
Elavil	amitriptyline	10–50 mg	12–24 hours

Antidepressants (*continued*)

Pamelor	nortriptyline	10–50 mg	16–90 hours
Sinequan	doxepin	10–50 mg	17–50 hours
Remeron	mirtazapine	15–30 mg	25–40 hours

Antipsychotics

| Seroquel | quetiapine | 25–50 mg | 6 hours |

Melatonin analogues

| Rozerem | ramelteon | 8 mg | 1–2½ hours |

Antihistamine

| Benadryl | diphenhydramine | 25–50 mg | 2–8 hours |

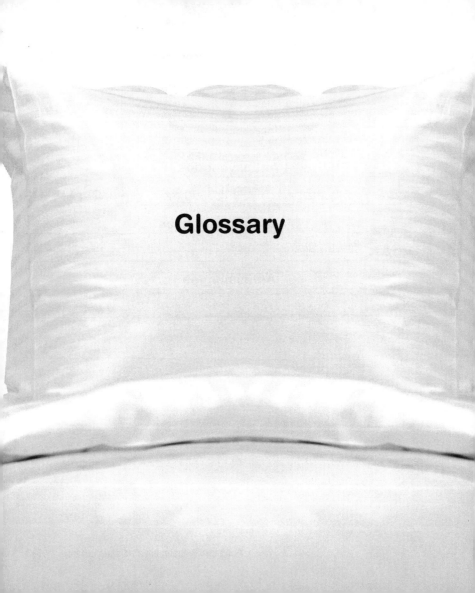

Glossary

Acupuncture: insertion of fine needles at specific points on the body for therapeutic purposes

Advanced Sleep Phase: a body clock shift in which there is a tendency to become sleepy early in the evening and awaken before dawn; compare Delayed Sleep Phase below

APAP: autoadjusting positive airway pressure

Apnea: absence of breathing during sleep for at least ten seconds

Bilevel positive airway pressure: a treatment for sleep apnea that utilizes different pressures for inspiration and expiration

Circadian rhythm: a daily (twenty-four-hour) pattern of biologic function such as the sleep-wake cycle

Cognitive behavioral therapy (CBT): techniques that allow people to deal with psychological problems and insomnia by recognizing and changing certain patterns of thought

Confusional arousal: a brief incomplete awakening from sleep

CPAP: continuous positive airway pressure, the primary treatment for obstructive sleep apnea

Delayed Sleep Phase: a body clock shift which turns people into night owls, creating the tendency for very late bedtimes and delayed awakenings in the morning

Drowsiness: transitional state between wakefulness and sleep

EEG: electroencephalogram, the instrument used to measure electrical activity in the brain

EMG: electromyogram; a diagnostic instrument used to measure muscle activity

Endorphins: endogenous substances produced in the human body with narcotic-like properties

EOG: electrooculogram; monitoring of eye movement during sleep (The EEG, EMG and EOG are used together to help physicians determine sleep stage.)

Epworth Sleepiness Scale: self-administered test which helps determine whether sleepiness is present. A score of 10 or greater on the Epworth Sleepiness Scale suggests a propensity to fall asleep in various situations

Fortune-telling error: the prediction that bad things will happen even though you have no good evidence that they will

GERD: Gastroesophageal Reflux Disease

HEPA filter: a high efficiency particulate air filter that can filter out unwanted particles in the air

Hypopnea: a decrease in airflow due to partial collapse of the airway during sleep

Hypnotics: sleep medications, commonly called sleeping pills

Insomnia: difficulty initiating or maintaining sleep

Melatonin: a hormone secreted by the pineal gland that plays a role in establishing the sleep-wake cycle; the amount decreases as people get older

Night terrors: also known as sleep terrors; episodes of apparent terror that can occur when the brain is partly awake and partly in non-REM sleep

Non-REM sleep: stages 1, 2, and 3 of sleep, the stages not associated with remembered dreaming

Parasomnia: broad term used to describe any unusual, abnormal, or unpleasant event which occurs during sleep

Periodic leg movement: involuntary leg movements in sleep that appear with a regular rhythm in intervals of 5 to 90 seconds in groups of at least four. These movements may be related to restless legs syndrome in some individuals

Reflux: the presence of corrosive acids in your esophagus originating from the stomach. Symptoms may include a burning sensation, cough, wheezing, shortness of breath, or a high-pitched sound during inspiration, known as stridor

REM sleep behavior disorder: a sleep disorder in which the normal muscle paralysis that occurs during REM sleep is absent, so the person has the capability of acting out dreams

REM sleep: Rapid Eye Movement sleep, the stage of sleep that is commonly associated with dreams we can remember

Rhinitis: inflammation of the nasal passage that leads to swelling and decreased airflow

Serotonin: a neurotransmitter in the brain known to play an important role in mood disturbances

Skeletal muscle paralysis: the condition in REM sleep in which most of your muscles cannot move

Sleep: a reversible state of unconsciousness; a biorhythm in synch with the light-dark cycle

Sleep architecture: the structure of sleep

Sleep hygiene: healthful practices that help you fall asleep and maintain restful sleep

Sleep state misperception: a perception that less time is spent in a sleep state than is actually the case

Sleep restriction: an insomnia treatment in which patients are instructed to go to bed much later than their desired bedtime

Sleepwalking: episodes occurring in non-REM sleep during which a person appears to be doing something purposeful, but remains asleep

Slow-wave sleep: commonly called "deep sleep," the most refreshing stage of sleep

TCM: Traditional Chinese Medicine; an alternative system to Western medicine that includes treatments such as massage, acupuncture, dietary therapy, and herbal medicine

Zeitgeiber: German for "time giver"; refers to light, noise, and other stimuli that provide cues to the brain during the sleep-wake cycle

Bibliography

Selected References and Websites

Alternative Therapies

American Botanical Council: *http://abc.herbalgram.org/site/PageServer*

American Council on Exercise: *www.acefitness.org*

Traditional Chinese Medicine: *www.tcmpage.com*

Dreams

Dreams: God's Forgotten Language, John A. Sanford, HarperOne, 1989.

Dreams and Healing, John A. Sanford, Paulist Press, 1988.

The Interpretation of Dreams, Sigmund Freud, Modern Library, 1994.

Sleep Medicine

The International Classification of Sleep Disorders Diagnostic and Coding Manual (Second Edition), American Academy of Sleep Medicine, Westchester IL, 2005.

Sleep Medicine: Essentials and Review, Teofilo Lee-Chiong, Oxford University Press, 2008.

Principles and Practice of Sleep Medicine 4th Edition, Kryger, M.H., Roth T., Dement, W.C. Saunders, Philadelphia, 2005.

Sleep Medicine, Lee-Chiong T.F., Sateia, M.J., Carskadon, M.A. Hanley and Belfus, Inc. Philadelphia, 2002.

Index